Starting & Your Own Physical Therapy Practice

A Practical Guide for the Rookie Entrepreneur

Samuel H. Esterson, PT, MBA, DScPT

Assistant Clinical Professor
University of Maryland–Baltimore
School of Medicine
Department of Physical Therapy
and Rehabilitation Science

◆

Esterson & Associates Physical Therapy, PA
Baltimore, Maryland

JONES AND BARTLETT PUBLISHERS
Sudbury, Massachusetts
BOSTON   TORONTO   LONDON   SINGAPORE

World Headquarters

Jones and Bartlett
Publishers
40 Tall Pine Drive
Sudbury, MA 01776
978-443-5000
info@jbpub.com
www.jbpub.com

Jones and Bartlett
Publishers Canada
6339 Ormindale Way
Mississauga, ON L5V 1J2
CANADA

Jones and Bartlett
Publishers International
Barb House, Barb Mews
London W6 7PA
UK

Library of Congress Cataloging-in-Publication Data

Esterson, Samuel H.
  Starting & managing your own physical therapy practice : a practical guide for the
rookie entrepreneur / Samuel H. Esterson.
    p. ; cm.
  Includes bibliographical references and index.
  ISBN 0-7637-2631-1 (pbk.)
  1. Physical therapy—Practice.
  [DNLM: 1. Physical Therapy (Specialty)—organization & administration. 2. Practice
Management. WB 460 E79s 2004] I. Title: Starting and managing your own physical
therapy practice. II. Title.
  RM705.E815 2004
  615.8'2'068—dc22

6048   2004007892

Production Credits
Executive Editor: Dave Cella
Production Director: Amy Rose
Production Editor: Tracey Chapman
Production Assistant: Rachel Rossi
Production Coordination: Jennifer Bagdigian
Associate Editor: Kylah Goodfellow McNeill
Editorial Assistant: Lisa Gordon
Manufacturing Buyer: Amy Bacus
Text Design and Composition: Auburn Associates, Inc.
Cover Design: Diana Coe
Printing and Binding: Malloy, Inc.
Cover Printing: Malloy, Inc.

Printed in the United States of America
08 07 06   10 9 8 7 6 5 4 3

Foreword

For a faculty member, observing the growth, development, and productivity of former students over the years is always a pleasure. Samuel Esterson is one of those former students. Since graduating, he has consistently improved his skills and expanded his knowledge. In his practice as a physical therapist, he always strives for excellence in his endeavors, whether it be as a clinician in a rehabilitation institution, a mentor and clinician in a hospital setting, the owner of a private practice, or a post-professional student at the MBA or Doctoral level. He has now taken his years of experience in private practice and has come forth with an invaluable, yet very practical, resource for those who want to start their own private physical therapy practice.

There is no doubt that the venues in which physical therapists practice have changed over time, particularly over the last 20 years. In 1983, almost 42% of physical therapists practiced in hospital facilities, while approximately 15% were in private practices. Now, almost 30% are in private practice and a little over 13% are in acute care facilities. These changes in private practice make this book all the more important for both the physical therapist starting a private practice and the physical therapist student.

This is indeed a "how-to" book. The author draws upon his own varied experiences developing his own private practices, as well as his formalized business training. He begins by having the practitioner analyze the motives for embarking upon a private practice, and then takes the practitioner through all the steps of establishing the framework of the practice and the costs, presenting needed banking information, developing the business and strategic plans, ascertaining what outside expertise will be needed, setting up the practice, and handling all of the areas related to Medicare/Medicaid, other insurance plans, marketing, advertising, coding, accounting, and staffing.

In an extremely organized approach, and with the inclusion of many practical resources available through the Web and many sample forms, the author has managed to present a great deal of material in an easily understandable format. Attention-getting symbols throughout the book alert the physical therapist practitioner to great ideas, to stop and think, to save information, to ask the lawyer or accountant, and to beware and seek help.

This book enables the physical therapist about to embark upon a private practice venture to fulfill her dreams and to do so in an orderly, structured way. Wasted hours and many mistakes will be avoided by using this book as a personal private practice mentor.

Marilyn Moffat, PT, PhD, FAPTA, CSCS
Professor, Physical Therapy Department
New York University

Preface

Let's be very clear about something: Starting a private practice can be a daunting task—but it's well worth the effort. Samuel Esterson's book *Starting & Managing Your Own Physical Therapy Practice: A Practical Guide for the Rookie Entrepreneur* can make the entire process a lot less challenging. Over the past 20 years, I have helped over 100 physical therapists start their own practices. On several occasions, in several markets, I have also started my own private physical therapy practice. In each case, this book would have been very helpful in the process. The profession has waited long enough for such an easy-to-read, simple-to-follow "How To" book to guide the therapist to open and run the office of his or her dreams. Many clinicians will reap success from using this text as their guide.

Dr. Samuel Esterson is well prepared to help you and me start our practices. As a private practitioner for 20 years, an educator, mentor, and serious "student" of marketing and business management (the "MBA" sure was helpful!), Sam offers practical, focused, and meaningful suggestions for success in private practice.

The actual entrepreneurial path you take will be unique to you. I find the diversity of possible pathways to be one of the most attractive aspects of captaining my own ship. You will too. There are, however, some tasks that all new businesses (that is what you will be—a new business) must tackle. Sam addresses many of these, from how to structure your business, to budgeting, marketing, and even why you want to own your own business. Although the entire process is quite complex, Sam helps keep things in perspective and addresses the critical issues in a clear and even humorous manner. His step-by-step method will take you from your dream to the office's opening day with real examples, instructions, websites, and templates that one can use immediately and easily.

The time is ripe for those therapists with an entrepreneurial spirit to start their own practice. ***Starting & Managing Your Own Physical Therapy Practice*** will help the reader in the pursuit of his or her practice dream. I recommend this book to every practitioner who is starting or even considering starting a practice. You need a variety of experts to help you—Samuel Esterson is one of those experts. Read and enjoy.

Peter Kovacek, PT, MSA
Owner, Kovacek Management Services, Inc.
1st Choice Physical Therapy, LLC
In Home Rehab, LLC
Harper Woods, MI

Dedications and Appreciations

This book that you are holding in your hands is the product of many hours of planning, thought, dedication, and diligence. It would have never come to light if not for the encouragement and support of my wife, Malka. I am indebted to her for her patience, fortitude, and encouragement for this and all my other projects and I dedicate this book to her.

To my three sons, Yonah, Elan, and Ari: You are my pride and joy. I thank you for giving me the time and space to work on this project. I appreciate the confidence you have in me, and I am likewise very proud of all your wonderful accomplishments. It is with gratitude that I also dedicate this book to you three.

I am indebted to Dr. Leslie B. Glickman, my doctoral advisor, mentor, colleague, and friend for her editing skills, late night e-mail critiques, and valuable advice along the way. Her contagious energy, passion, and drive for bigger and better things gave me the extra push to take this project to completion.

Many thanks to Peter Kovacek, one of our profession's foremost business management gurus, for his encouragement and peer review of the manuscript.

Table of Contents

Introduction

Wouldn't it be a snap if all it took to open and run a successful private practice would be a diploma from physical therapy school and a few bucks? Wouldn't it be terrific just to hang out a shingle with your name on it and all you would have to do would be to hold off the multitudes of potential patients from tearing your door down seeking your expertise? Wouldn't it be a breeze if you could just say a few magic words and suddenly the office would be fully appointed with state-of-the-art equipment and furniture, and patients would just flow in and out, pleased and satisfied with anything and everything you did for them? Wouldn't it be a cinch if you never had to know about contracts, taxes, referral sources, receivables, payables, liability insurance, and managed care organizations? Unfortunately, those who believe the old adage, "build it and they will come," have it all wrong. In this day and age, healthcare professionals are setting themselves up for a simple and rapid demise if they don't contemplate, plan, execute, reassess, and appropriately adjust their performance, whether opening a new practice or expanding a current one.

A Note to the Reader

The chapters ahead include icons to emphasize valuable information, to proceed with caution, to get help, and to point out words of wisdom. The writing style is casual and notes the author's experience to emphasize a point. This style was chosen for ease of reading and application of information versus the formal style of most academic texts.

As Luck Would Have It

I used to hear that whenever a certain businessman was obviously successful, people remarked that he was lucky: He was in the right place at the right time, his father gave him all the money so how could he lose, or that he just had a golden touch. My definition of luck is having a vision to initially see an existing opportunity, and then grabbing it. Most everyone goes around on the same merry-go-round of life. There are gold rings to grab at many posts along the way. The real entrepreneur (see ahead for the definition of this seemingly French word) knows where to look for the proverbial ring, takes the proper risks in planning for the most appropriate time and place to grab the ring, and then finally reaches out clearly and grasps it. Interestingly, the entrepreneur doesn't stop there. His next step is to look for more rings, better rings, more expansive or easier-to-reach rings, knowing that the rings don't stay valuable forever and that new and different types of rings are necessary to keep his business going. That is what separates the entrepreneur from the common businessman or working-class stiff.

Dream On

The difference between fulfilling your greatest dream and living your worst nightmare is basic: business education, proper planning, and a passion to succeed. Those of us who want to paddle our own boat instead of floating along, swabbing the deck on someone else's yacht, have to know a good deal of business management, marketing, accounting, and legal navigation. Many of us have the passion but not the experience. So where do we go from here?

About This Book

You are probably thinking, "but how do I start this journey?" This text was written to give the *rookie* entrepreneur physical therapist a business advantage over the competition. Our professional education gave us a mere glimpse at what business is all about, but if we are putting our name, reputation, and pocketbook on the line, we need to know just how to do it right the first time. This book offers insight into the hows, whats, and wheres of private business, and gives the practitioner enough information and insight to veer him in the proper direction. It is not a business bible, nor does it attempt to answer every business question you, as an entrepreneur, may have. There are tons of books on the market discussing starting a small business, but none address the special requirements and needs we as physical therapists have. This book is a guide map, a tool developed to open your eyes to what is necessary to open and run your own successful practice. Insights and ideas are taken from my 20-plus years of professional and business practice in many venues from large hospital facilities and corporate therapy groups to private practice enterprises.

The text is divided into 15 chapters. The sequence is designed to lead you through the planning, executing, and outcome assessment phases of management in a step-by-step fashion. Chapter 1 asks you to take a look at yourself, your talents, and your motivation to become a private practitioner. It discusses the reasons for opening your own practice and suggests avenues to explore whether or not you have the wherewithal and adrenaline to cut it as an entrepreneur. Are you ready? Do you have what it takes to put in way more than eight hours a day? If so, Chapter 2 discusses the importance of picking a company name and discusses the advantages and disadvantages of the different business structures you may choose. The section ends with a description of the first magic number you must obtain before going any further in business. Determining what everything will cost and budgeting appropriately is covered in Chapter 3. Setting up your finances and bank account is covered in Chapter 4. Chapter 5 teaches you how to turn your ideas into reality by creating a mission and vision statement, leading you into the business planning stage. Chapter 6 identifies the list of advisors and team members you'll need to make your dream happen and avoid aggravation when you need a helping hand. It identifies the members of what I call your "dream team," those professionals who will help you make the most cost-effective, legal, and intelligent decisions about your new venture. Chapter 7 gets into the nitty-gritty of establishing the business, the phase of "setting up shop."

Medicare is sometimes called the *insurance giant* of reimbursement. Chapter 8 explains what Medicare is and why it is important for you to become a credentialed provider with the *giant*. Marketing, also called *drumming up business*, is probably the most time-consuming and difficult part of keeping a practice going, and is detailed in Chapter 9. I'll save you time and money in Chapter 10's discussion about advertising and promotional printing. I have even included samples in the Appendix of each form I use. In addition, this chapter discusses how to promote your name and image with marketing, including using website technology. Chapter 11 describes the *payer mix* and the importance of not putting your reimbursement eggs in one carrier's basket. In that section, I have also covered HMO, PPO, and IPA definitions and descriptions. Chapter 12 teaches you the billing game, that is, how you bill and what you can expect to be paid for your services. Your accountant will throw all kinds of numbers at you. To keep you informed and teach you the basics of financial fitness and fiscal responsibility, Chapter 13 provides you with a table of the various state and federal taxes you'll be responsible to pay monthly, quarterly, and yearly. With all the revenue you are already bringing in, you'll need staff to help you continue to grow. Your employees are your most valuable commodities. Chapter 14 tells you how to find employees, how to pick the best of the crop, and how to take care of them once you have them. The importance of the employee handbook is included. A sample employee manual table of contents can be found in the Appendix. Lastly, Chapter 15 teaches you how to assess your own business performance and outcomes, answering your question: Is everything working OK? Outcome research is necessary to inform the owner if he is doing well, and how much better he can expect to do by making financial changes, juggling the staffing, and/or making modifications in procedures. The Appendix is chock-full of sample forms, diagrams, illustrations, and other resources to start and build your practice, a list of state insurance carriers, a sample pro-forma budget, and an opening day checklist. Finally, at the close of each chapter, a few wise words will jump-start you to think of various business-related concepts.

Attention-Grabbing Symbols Used in This Book

These little cartoons are used to grab your attention throughout this book. They will focus your attention on important, sometimes lifesaving, matters in business.

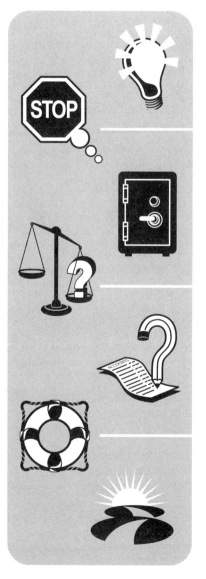

A tip, a great idea, or a way to save you time, effort, and cash.

Stop and think twice about this. It will save you from aggravation later.

Valuable information that you should keep and not forget

Ask your lawyer

Ask your accountant

Beware: it looks easier than it really is. **Get help.**

Wise words to enlighten you in your path to success

CHAPTER 1

Are You Sure You Want to Open a Practice?

The Entrepreneurial Physical Therapist

First, let's define the term entrepreneur. According to Merriam-Webster Online, an entrepreneur is one who organizes, manages, and assumes the risks of a business or enterprise (from the French, *entreprendre*, to undertake). The entrepreneur is a mover and shaker, is enthusiastic, welcomes a challenge, is a risk taker, is creative and innovative, and is not averse to change. Entrepreneurs are persistent and demand as much of themselves as they do of others. They are born leaders and motivators. Entrepreneurs have a passion for their dreams and don't easily take "no" for an answer. They calculate their risks and plan their moves carefully. Entrepreneurs learn from their mistakes and don't give up. They see the glass as half full while others perceive it as half empty. Entrepreneurs see opportunity when others see potential failure. Traits like these are not common, but if you have a large combination of any of these characteristics and have an interest in determining your own destiny, with the right tools and planning, your success is within closer reach than you think.

Years back, anyone who opened a business may have been considered an entrepreneur by virtue of the fact that they had the sheer *chutzpah* (guts) to open a business when others dared not. It wasn't until the 1980s, when university business schools began studying the subject, that entrepreneurship was seen as an outlook and a passion, a way to look at opportunity as a road map to success. Even if you don't possess all the typical entrepreneurial traits, understanding how the entrepreneur ticks gives you insight into the opportunistic mindset. Business savvy is not equated with academic prowess. It is a process of planning, executing, jockeying for position, regrouping, and starting again. This book is written to give YOU the basics of this process. Do you have the drive, stick-to-itiveness, and dedication to make it happen? Do you have what it takes to seize the opportunity as it presents itself? Are you the budding entrepreneur? If so, let's get started.

Should I Really Open My Own Practice?

 If you are thinking, "Yeah, I want to be my own boss" because you are tired of taking orders from your manager and hate when he tells you when to take lunch, forget about branching out on your own. Being your own boss is more about satisfying others than about being an independent businessman. Once you open your own business, you must satisfy four different customer groups: your patients, your referral sources, your staff, and your patients' payers (insurance companies). They are your new bosses, and their needs differ from yours. You must take good care of these four groups of customers and keep them happy if you want to see success. They are like the torches of fire that the juggler must constantly keep in motion and in harmony, lest the juggler himself gets burned. If any one of your four new bosses falls out of synchronous harmony, you too may get burned. So, with that in mind, along with constant worries about making payroll, rent, and supply order payments; keeping the schedule flowing smoothly; having enough new referrals to fill your staff's daily log; developing personnel and procedure manuals; contracting with every Tom, Dick, and Harry insurance carrier around; and other associated ulcer-producing tasks, why on earth did you say you wanted to be your own boss? Phew!

What Motivates You?

Look in the mirror. Do you see someone with a real desire to succeed, one with the fortitude and drive to make it happen? Why do you want to start your own practice? Hopefully, the words are flowing off your tongue right now. Here are common reasons people decide to enter private practice:

◆ **Flexibility:** They want to determine the amount of time they dedicate to work and home life.
◆ **Earning potential:** They want greater compensation for working harder and longer hours.
◆ **Creativity:** They enjoy bettering the status quo.
◆ **Control:** They want to be their own boss and control their own destiny.
◆ **Adventure:** They like taking risks.
◆ **Challenge:** They thrive on prioritizing and balancing their lives.
◆ **Innovation:** They like to create something from nothing.
◆ **Pride:** They delight in their own accomplishments.
◆ **Status:** They seek the status of being "in charge" and making decisions.
◆ **Leadership:** They are leaders and builders.
◆ **Managing:** They are comfortable delegating tasks to others and supervising them.
◆ **Independence:** They value their freedom and its benefits.
◆ **Non-risk averse:** They love challenges.

Do You **Have** What It Takes?

Many self-help business texts address this issue more extensively, but, in a nutshell, how do you know if you do *have* what it takes to start your own practice? Looking at your own personality inventory is a good start:

◆ **What is your work style?**
◆ **What and who motivates you?**
◆ **Are you a planner and a doer?**
◆ **Are you a risk taker and a self-initiator?**
◆ **What kind of interpersonal skills do you have?**
◆ **Are you a leader and a motivator of others?**
◆ **Are you insightful and see an opportunity others may miss?**
◆ **Are you a problem solver and do you have business savvy?**
◆ **How well do you work with others?**
◆ **Do others look up to you?**
◆ **Are you hard working and goal-directed?**
◆ **Are you persistent and dynamic?**
◆ **Do you easily take "no" for an answer?**

These and other traits are descriptive of someone who has the potential of starting and building a successful business. Be honest. If the majority of these traits describe you, you may have what it takes.

To SWOT or Not?

SWOT stands for Strengths, Weaknesses, Opportunities, and Threats. Critical self-assessment using SWOT analysis is a helpful tool in deciding whether you have what it takes to make it on your own or not. It will be a challenging experience to define and apply these four words to you. Who among us cannot rattle off our strengths and perhaps the opportunities we see in opening our own enterprise? On the other side of the matrix, SWOT analysis forces you to verbalize your weaknesses and threats, two areas most people shudder to admit. If the Weaknesses and Threats areas of your SWOT overwhelmingly outweigh the Strengths and Opportunities, **watch out**! Perhaps you should reconsider your idea or the timing of your plan, or look more optimistically at yourself, or ask someone whose opinion you value to give you objective input (not your mother or spouse).

The following table shows a sample SWOT analysis for a physical therapist with five years of clinical experience in a community hospital outpatient department contemplating opening his own practice:

STRENGTHS	WEAKNESSES
◆ Reputation as a senior therapist ◆ Outgoing personality ◆ Certified Clinical Specialist ◆ Doctoral degree ◆ Relationship with hospital physicians ◆ Past marketing experience	◆ No prior business experience ◆ Moderate level clinical experience ◆ Limited finances for start-up ◆ Beginning with Medicare and commercial carrier credentialing only
OPPORTUNITIES	**THREATS**
◆ Niche market TMJ specialty ◆ Location adjacent to hospital and several dentists' offices ◆ Potential to work with school teams ◆ Managed care participation	◆ Competition of existing private practices, hospital outpatient departments, and POPTS ◆ Managed care panel potential lock out

Know Your Entrepreneurial Talents

After performing your SWOT, it is useful to have some insight into your entrepreneurial traits and strengths. This information can advise you about some areas in which you may want to ask for assistance or advice and other areas where you have particular strengths.

 There are several online assessments that can help you determine your entrepreneurial talents, including your strengths and weaknesses. Once you know them, there are two ways to deal with them—you can either improve your skills in the areas where you're weak (by taking a class in marketing, for example), or hire an employee to handle these aspects of business (for instance, hiring a marketing rep). Check out these sites for further information:

◆ *http://www.wd.gc.ca*
  The Western Diversification "Am I an Entrepreneur?": Self-assessment Quiz. Do you have what it takes to be an entrepreneur? This tool gives you an opportunity to compare yourself with successful entrepreneurs and business owners on some key traits and characteristics. It also helps to determine your entrepreneurial qualities and gain an insight into your own distinctive entrepreneurial style.

◆ *http://www.navis.gr/manager/entrepre.htm*
  This assessment tests your Entrepreneurial Quotient. Common characteristics in areas such as family background, childhood experiences, core values, personalities, and more turn up time and time again in studies of entrepreneurs. The brief online test does not claim to measure your future success, but it may show you where you excel and where you need to improve to help make your business soar.

◆ *http://www.career-intelligence.com/assessment/ personality/entrepreneurs_checklist.html*
  Sure, talent and a great idea will help you get started, but having an "entrepreneurial personality" may help you make it big in the long run. Most successful entrepreneurs are enterprising, resourceful, and energetic. They live for the challenge of crea-

tive problem solving, decision making, and juggling their options. Try this test online and see if you are a born leader and have the ability to inspire, persuade, and motivate others.

♦ *http://www.bizmove.com/other/quiz.htm*

In considering opening your own business of any sort, one of the first questions you should answer for yourself is "Am I the type?" Since you will be your most important employee and take the lead in every aspect of the business, it is important that you rate yourself objectively, appraise your strengths and your weaknesses, and then be honest with yourself by acknowledging your own shortcomings. The results of this assessment will indicate to what extent you have the personal traits important to a business proprietor.

♦ *http://uwadmnweb.uwyo.edu/RanchRecr/handbook/*
Entrepreneurship_test.htm

Check out your personal background, behavior patterns, and lifestyle, and compare them to the qualities most entrepreneurs display. The questions were designed to represent various characteristics that studies have shown entrepreneurs tend to exhibit.

♦ *http://www.potentielentrepreneur.ca/client/*
questionnairesection1en.asp

The Business Development Bank of Canada Entrepreneurial Self-Assessment test assesses your entrepreneurial spirit. By completing this online questionnaire on attitude and lifestyle, you can assess how consistent your character is with that of proven successful entrepreneurs.

♦ *http://www.small-business.co.il*

So you say you have the interest and drive to be an entrepreneur but do not feel that you have all the desirable traits of a true mover and shaker. Don't despair. Another slick and outstanding self-assessment quiz to see how you measure up to other potential entrepreneurs is "The Entrepreneur Test." This test assesses your strengths and weaknesses and allows you to acknowledge your weaknesses. By knowing your weak areas, you can compensate for your deficiencies by either retraining yourself or hiring someone with the necessary skills you may lack. The questions in this test indicate to what extent you have the personal traits to become a successful proprietor.

What Is My Goal in All of This?

Most people when asked this question would reply "to make money, of course, and to be highly regarded in the professional community." The definition of success varies from person to person, but the definition of the business goal should remain rock steady—to consistently increase the value of the company. Value can be increased in several ways: by increasing sales (revenues), that is, the number of patient visits per day in your clinic; by decreasing expenses; and by decreasing the adjustments to gross sales, that is, how much money is not received by you due to insurance write-offs, bad debt, poor collections, and the like. Communication is a big slice of the success pie.

As mentioned earlier, starting your own practice means changing your time availability for patient care convenience, for meeting with potential referring practitioners, for business conferences with your accountant or attorney, and other time-consuming parts of life that those not in private industry may not understand or agree with. Your spouse, family, children, friends, and business colleagues should be informed of your decision to go out on your own and how your time commitment priorities may be changing. In short, it all depends on you. Are you searching for a better, potentially more lucrative, and greater satisfying job? Do you feel that stirring inside that tells you to "go do it" as opposed to taking an antacid? Are you willing to make a calculated risk to make more of yourself and your profession? If so, I am ready to give you the guidelines and tips for starting your own practice. If not, perhaps you are just not ready yet or you have other priorities. Whenever you're ready, the following pages are here for you as an easy method of navigating the complicated paths of opening your own practice. Read on!

Can I Try It First to See If I Like It?

To jump in with both feet, you will immediately give up your regular job, work longer hours, compromise home life to some extent or another, and enter a roller coaster of emotions. What a thrill! Can you try out some part-time independent work while still at your regular job? Can you pick up some private patients on the side after your regular work hours at the hospital or rehabilitation center? If so, it is a great way to taste the world of private enterprise. You have the best of both worlds and can ponder your comfort level. You can estimate what additional income you can generate and live on, how to maximize your productivity while still keeping the business end even, and experiencing a portion of private business while not taking the full risk of jumping in all at once. Even if you choose to test the waters first, keep reading. You will still need to know the risks of private enterprise and how to avoid potential pitfalls even as a part-time independent practitioner.

A Decalogue of Canons for Observation in Practical Life:

1. Never put off until tomorrow what you can do today.
2. Never trouble another for what you can do yourself.
3. Never spend money before you have it.
4. Never buy what you do not want, because it is cheap; it will be dear to you.
5. Pride costs us more than hunger, thirst, and cold.
6. We never repent of having eaten too little.
7. Nothing is troublesome that we do willingly.
8. How much pain have cost us the evils which never have happened.
9. Take things away by their smooth handle.
10. When angry, count to ten before you speak; if very angry, a hundred.

—Thomas Jefferson

CHAPTER 2

Establishing the Structural Framework

What's in a Name?

The Name Game—It's a game we have to play to figure out who we are and come up with a way to convince our customers to remember us. Is it better to have a corporate name or use your own name? It just depends. I have always been of the opinion that I am selling my name and expertise. My name is always on the line. The referring practitioner knows that he can call me personally when he has an issue or a special problem. The buck stops with me. I'm the man. I'm the owner. I'm the boss. With that said, shouldn't I think that Esterson & Associates Physical Therapy would be a plausible corporate name? Of course I do, and that's why it became the company's name. If I sell my name to the customers, all four of them, how could they forget me?

What's the down side? Well, the largest problem is that I can only treat a given number of patients a day. Like you, I have only 24 hours in each day. So as I grow, I add staff therapists and then more therapists and then more therapists. What happens then? The referring practitioners tell all their patients that they want Esterson himself to see them. Ouch! But, I can't manage to see 32 patients a day myself. What's the solution? All my staff therapists are encouraged to personally market referring practitioners, both current and potential referrers, with their own business cards using the corporate name but stating their names and titles as well.

 "I work with Sam," the therapist says. The referring practitioner matches the two and is happy to have his patients seen here. Every therapist is listed prominently on my letterhead. I make sure that the exterior door sign reads Esterson & Associates Physical Therapy, listing my own name along with each practitioner I employ. We all have associates, don't we? Associates are people we empirically trust and rely upon. I am determined that each of my staff develops a close enough relationship with our customers so they are likewise known and trusted, making it easy for the referring practitioners to send their patients our way to see the boss or any of his associates. By advertising each staff therapist's name, they have a sense of pride in our practice and feel ownership for the services we provide. I have seen the staff bond together as a working team with a special cohesiveness and feeling of anticipated cooperation. Most importantly, having every therapist's name displayed on our door relays to our patients that we are all equally licensed and qualified to care for each patient who crosses our doorstep. This lessens the potential of a patient objecting to the possibility of multiple clinicians providing care for them.

On the flip side of the coin, some owners believe that they can avoid this confusion and headache by naming the corporation with a cute, easily remembered, location-based name like Hands-On Therapy Associates of Hampden, Tricounty Physical Therapy, Annapolis Eldercare Rehabilitation, or Harford County Physical Therapy, among others. When looking at a location name, one never knows who is running the show. My personal bias says it is much harder marketing a location versus a name. I am not yet convinced that even highly educated healthcare providers can remember more than one name at a time. In the case of Esterson & Associates Physical Therapy, it is at least assumed that in some capacity, a guy named Esterson will be involved with the referred patient. He may treat the patient or at least greet that patient, having some level of contact with him. If you do choose to go with your own name, make it your business to see and be seen in your clinic. Introduce yourself to as many patients and family members as you can during your workday. Let every patient know that they are in the best hands around (no pun intended). Train your staff in these methods so patients who may see more than one therapist during their experience at your clinic will feel equally comfortable with all your staff therapists. In any event, before you move to the next step and tell Uncle Sam about yourself, you need to identify yourself professionally.

What's Your Structure: Corporate or Solo?

 Surely your attorney will lead you through this decision, but it is important to at least be familiar with the various business structure possibilities. There are three basic business organizational structures: sole proprietorships, partnerships, and corporations. There are subclasses under each structure that may or may not apply to your specific situation.

In *legalese*, a language you will never fully understand and will always need to pay an attorney to fully comprehend, the main difference between the corporate structures is the extent to which the law protects your business in the event of a business disaster. The term that describes the protection that a corporation affords is called the "corporate veil." A corporation, once established, is an entity all itself and as the "business owner," you, for all intents and purposes, work for and are paid by this separate entity. This so-called "veil" protects you from financial and civil liabilities. Don't be fooled! The corporate veil does not shield you from professional injuries you may cause or damages that may befall you. For those, be sure your malpractice premiums are paid up.

Here is some detail on each legal structure to help you discuss the pros and cons of each with your legal advisor:

- ◆ **I fly solo:** The *Sole Proprietor* opens his doors and services to his customers using his own name on the door and on his checks. It is simple and cheap to create this business structure and any and all profits flow directly to the owner. For the Internal Revenue Service (IRS) to track your sales and earnings, you must file an SS-4 form for a Tax Identification Number (TIN) (see pages 12 and 13). The down side of this arrangement is if you get sued by a customer for any reason, even for something one of your employees did, you have no veil, no legal protection, and can lose anything and everything you've worked so hard to achieve.
- ◆ **Let's do it together:** The *Partnership* arrangement is like a marriage. Everything is shared and divided according to a written

Form **SS-4** (Rev. December 2001) Department of the Treasury Internal Revenue Service	**Application for Employer Identification Number** (For use by employers, corporations, partnerships, trusts, estates, churches, government agencies, Indian tribal entities, certain individuals, and others.) ▶ See separate instructions for each line. ▶ Keep a copy for your records.	EIN OMB No. 1545-0003

Type or print clearly.

1 Legal name of entity (or individual) for whom the EIN is being requested

2 Trade name of business (if different from name on line 1) | **3** Executor, trustee, "care of" name

4a Mailing address (room, apt., suite no. and street, or P.O. box) | **5a** Street address (if different) (Do not enter a P.O. box.)

4b City, state, and ZIP code | **5b** City, state, and ZIP code

6 County and state where principal business is located

7a Name of principal officer, general partner, grantor, owner, or trustor | **7b** SSN, ITIN, or EIN

8a Type of entity (check only one box)
- ☐ Sole proprietor (SSN) _____
- ☐ Partnership
- ☐ Corporation (enter form number to be filed) ▶ _____
- ☐ Personal service corp.
- ☐ Church or church-controlled organization
- ☐ Other nonprofit organization (specify) ▶ _____
- ☐ Other (specify) ▶

- ☐ Estate (SSN of decedent) _____
- ☐ Plan administrator (SSN) _____
- ☐ Trust (SSN of grantor) _____
- ☐ National Guard ☐ State/local government
- ☐ Farmers' cooperative ☐ Federal government/military
- ☐ REMIC ☐ Indian tribal governments/enterprises
- Group Exemption Number (GEN) ▶

8b If a corporation, name the state or foreign country (if applicable) where incorporated | State | Foreign country

9 Reason for applying (check only one box)
- ☐ Started new business (specify type) ▶ _____
- ☐ Hired employees (Check the box and see line 12.)
- ☐ Compliance with IRS withholding regulations
- ☐ Other (specify) ▶

- ☐ Banking purpose (specify purpose) ▶ _____
- ☐ Changed type of organization (specify new type) ▶ _____
- ☐ Purchased going business
- ☐ Created a trust (specify type) ▶ _____
- ☐ Created a pension plan (specify type) ▶ _____

10 Date business started or acquired (month, day, year) | **11** Closing month of accounting year

12 First date wages or annuities were paid or will be paid (month, day, year). Note: If applicant is a withholding agent, enter date income will first be paid to nonresident alien. (month, day, year) . . . . ▶

13 Highest number of employees expected in the next 12 months. Note: If the applicant does not expect to have any employees during the period, enter "-0-." . . . . ▶ | Agricultural | Household | Other

14 Check one box that best describes the principal activity of your business. ☐ Health care & social assistance ☐ Wholesale–agent/broker
- ☐ Construction ☐ Rental & leasing ☐ Transportation & warehousing ☐ Accommodation & food service ☐ Wholesale–other ☐ Retail
- ☐ Real estate ☐ Manufacturing ☐ Finance & insurance ☐ Other (specify)

15 Indicate principal line of merchandise sold; specific construction work done; products produced; or services provided.

16a Has the applicant ever applied for an employer identification number for this or any other business? . . . . . ☐ Yes ☐ No
Note: If "Yes," please complete lines 16b and 16c.

16b If you checked "Yes" on line 16a, give applicant's legal name and trade name shown on prior application if different from line 1 or 2 above.
Legal name ▶ Trade name ▶

16c Approximate date when, and city and state where, the application was filed. Enter previous employer identification number if known.
Approximate date when filed (mo., day, year) | City and state where filed | Previous EIN

Third Party Designee	Complete this section only if you want to authorize the named individual to receive the entity's EIN and answer questions about the completion of this form.	
	Designee's name	Designee's telephone number (include area code) ( )
	Address and ZIP code	Designee's fax number (include area code) ( )

Under penalties of perjury, I declare that I have examined this application, and to the best of my knowledge and belief, it is true, correct, and complete. | Applicant's telephone number (include area code) ( )

Name and title (type or print clearly) ▶

Signature ▶ Date ▶ | Applicant's fax number (include area code) ( )

For Privacy Act and Paperwork Reduction Act Notice, see separate instructions. Cat. No. 16055N Form **SS-4** (Rev. 12-2001)

Do I Need an EIN?

File Form SS-4 if the applicant entity does not already have an EIN but is required to show an EIN on any return, statement, or other document.[1] See also the separate instructions for each line on Form SS-4.

IF the applicant...	AND...	THEN...
Started a new business	Does not currently have (nor expect to have) employees	Complete lines 1, 2, 4a–6, 8a, and 9–16c.
Hired (or will hire) employees, including household employees	Does not already have an EIN	Complete lines 1, 2, 4a–6, 7a–b (if applicable), 8a, 8b (if applicable), and 9–16c.
Opened a bank account	Needs an EIN for banking purposes only	Complete lines 1–5b, 7a–b (if applicable), 8a, 9, and 16a–c.
Changed type of organization	Either the legal character of the organization or its ownership changed (e.g., you incorporate a sole proprietorship or form a partnership)[2]	Complete lines 1–16c (as applicable).
Purchased a going business[3]	Does not already have an EIN	Complete lines 1–16c (as applicable).
Created a trust	The trust is other than a grantor trust or an IRA trust[4]	Complete lines 1–16c (as applicable).
Created a pension plan as a plan administrator[5]	Needs an EIN for reporting purposes	Complete lines 1, 2, 4a–6, 8a, 9, and 16a–c.
Is a foreign person needing an EIN to comply with IRS withholding regulations	Needs an EIN to complete a Form W-8 (other than Form W-8ECI), avoid withholding on portfolio assets, or claim tax treaty benefits[6]	Complete lines 1–5b, 7a–b (SSN or ITIN optional), 8a–9, and 16a–c.
Is administering an estate	Needs an EIN to report estate income on Form 1041	Complete lines 1, 3, 4a–b, 8a, 9, and 16a–c.
Is a withholding agent for taxes on non-wage income paid to an alien (i.e., individual, corporation, or partnership, etc.)	Is an agent, broker, fiduciary, manager, tenant, or spouse who is required to file Form 1042, Annual Withholding Tax Return for U.S. Source Income of Foreign Persons	Complete lines 1, 2, 3 (if applicable), 4a–5b, 7a–b (if applicable), 8a, 9, and 16a–c.
Is a state or local agency	Serves as a tax reporting agent for public assistance recipients under Rev. Proc. 80-4, 1980-1 C.B. 581[7]	Complete lines 1, 2, 4a–5b, 8a, 9, and 16a–c.
Is a single-member LLC	Needs an EIN to file Form 8832, Classification Election, for filing employment tax returns, or for state reporting purposes[8]	Complete lines 1–16c (as applicable).
Is an S corporation	Needs an EIN to file Form 2553, Election by a Small Business Corporation[9]	Complete lines 1–16c (as applicable).

[1] For example, a sole proprietorship or self-employed farmer who establishes a qualified retirement plan, or is required to file excise, employment, alcohol, tobacco, or firearms returns, must have an EIN. A partnership, corporation, REMIC (real estate mortgage investment conduit), nonprofit organization (church, club, etc.), or farmers' cooperative must use an EIN for any tax-related purpose even if the entity does not have employees.

[2] However, do not apply for a new EIN if the existing entity only (a) changed its business name, (b) elected on Form 8832 to change the way it is taxed (or is covered by the default rules), or (c) terminated its partnership status because at least 50% of the total interests in partnership capital and profits were sold or exchanged within a 12-month period. (The EIN of the terminated partnership should continue to be used. See Regulations section 301.6109-1(d)(2)(iii).)

[3] Do not use the EIN of the prior business unless you became the "owner" of a corporation by acquiring its stock.

[4] However, IRA trusts that are required to file Form 990-T, Exempt Organization Business Income Tax Return, must have an EIN.

[5] A plan administrator is the person or group of persons specified as the administrator by the instrument under which the plan is operated.

[6] Entities applying to be a Qualified Intermediary (QI) need a QI-EIN even if they already have an EIN. See Rev. Proc. 2000-12.

[7] See also Household employer on page 4. (Note: State or local agencies may need an EIN for other reasons, e.g., hired employees.)

[8] Most LLCs do not need to file Form 8832. See Limited liability company (LLC) on page 4 for details on completing Form SS-4 for an LLC.

[9] An existing corporation that is electing or revoking S corporation status should use its previously-assigned EIN.

agreement. The partnership is like a sole proprietorship owned by more than one person. Like the sole proprietor, there is no legal veil to protect the owners against lawsuits. All liability is passed to the partners. *Limited Partnerships* provide certain partners with a maximum financial liability commensurate with their investment. They are called limited partners and do not participate in day-to-day running of the company. The general partner runs the daily business matters and is in charge of the company from a legal standpoint.

◆ **Protect and Serve:** *Corporations* (also called C-corporations) are separate and distinct entities, similar to the creation of a new business life. Upon creation of the corporation, shareholders are issued stock. A board of directors elected by shareholders runs the corporation. The corporation, as a separate and distinct entity of its own, pays taxes on its annual profits, and passes monies to the shareholders, called dividends. The up side of incorporating your business is that with this structure, the corporation is responsible for its own financial and civil liabilities. The shareholders (owners) risk only the amount of money they initially invested into establishing the company. The other up side is that if you wish to expand some day and need to raise some money, you can sell more stock in the corporation and add those who choose to invest with you to the ownership of the company. There are caveats in this aspect related to professional corporations, including the fact that professional corporation structure is limited to the licensed professional offering specific benefits. Your legal advisor can fill you in on those details.

Here are two other subsets of the corporate structure that most private practices strongly consider:

◆ **Subchapter-S Corporation:** In this structure, you have the advantage of the corporate veil protecting you from financial and civil liabilities. Any and all profits flow directly into your personal bank account. This structure is not a pure separate entity in that it does not pay its own taxes, yet it has the other security and tax advantages of a conventional C-corporation.

◆ **Limited Liability Corporations (LLC):** The LLC is a relatively new type of entity that has only recently become available in all

50 states. Since it is so new, the laws among the various states differ somewhat in the treatment of an LLC. As a result, transactions
outside the state of formation by the LLC may be treated differently from transactions within the state of formation. This struc-
  • ture offers personal liability protection like the C-corporation and
allows profits to be funneled directly to the shareholders like the
Subchapter-S corporation.

The major difference between LLCs and S-corporations is
that the LLCs do not have the same restrictions regarding the
number of shareholders. S-corporations limit the number of
shareholders to 75 while LLCs can have unlimited shareholders. An LLC usually costs more to form and maintain than a
sole proprietorship or a general partnership. States may also
charge an initial formation fee and an annual fee, so check with
your state's secretary of state's office.

Where do you find out what's required in your state?
Though every state has its own rules and regulations, there is a
central place to start—the U.S. Small Business Administration
(SBA). Set your browser to *http://www.sba.gov* or call the SBA
Answer Desk at (800) 827-5722. The SBA can provide you with
helpful tips on starting a business, as well as links to each state's
website. Regarding the specifics about professionals forming
LLCs, The Consumer Media Group (*http://www.toolkit.cch.
com*) reports that all states, except California, now allow
professionals to form limited liability companies as well as
corporations.

All of these states impose on the LLC the same first condition imposed on the Professional Corporation or PC (i.e., all of
the owners must be licensed in the same profession). However,
curiously, many states do not impose the second condition on
LLCs (i.e., the condition that requires the business to use the
designation PC in its name).

In some states that do impose the second condition on LLCs,
the designation PLLC (Professional Limited Liability Company)
is used. In the states that do not impose the second condition, no
special identifiers are used other than LLC or PLLC.

If you are considering a professional LLC, inquire whether
the state in which you are forming the entity requires you to use

the designation PLLC in the business's name. In addition, it is always a good idea to check with your state chapter of the American Physical Therapy Association to determine if there are any special ethical rules or considerations regarding the operation of an LLC in your particular state.

TIN Is Not Something with Which to **Metal**

TIN stands for Tax Identification Number. It is also called an Employee Identification Number by the IRS, and every business needs one. Any and every business form you will fill out, from applying for Medicare providership to opening your bank account, will require this magic number. Fortunately, it's easy to get. All you need to do is obtain form SS-4 from the IRS website (www.irs.gov) or ask your accountant for one. The form asks you your corporate name, business name (if different), and your address. Complete the form, mail it in, and sit back and relax. In due time, the nine-digit TIN will be sent back by return mail. Alternately, you can obtain a TIN by calling the IRS toll free at (800) 829-1040.

Try not to become a man of success but rather a man of value.

—*Albert Einstein*

CHAPTER **3**

What's It All Cost?

How Do I Create a Budget for This Venture?

The most important concept that even experienced practice owners often overlook is that you must know what it costs you to do business. In the case of a physical therapy practice, you must know the actual expense to treat an average patient that crosses your threshold.

Cost Per Visit

Every finance and accounting textbook will show you how to calculate your cost of providing a product or service. Here is how I do it: Take your estimated total expenses for the year minus your profit (as an owner), add a staff therapist's salary to take the place of your profit you just excluded, and divide by the number of visits per year. This is a difficult calculation for a start-up venture because you do not yet know your actual expenses, but stay conservative in your guesstimate. Most practices see 12–18 visits per therapist per day. After subtracting a staff therapist's vacation time and holidays, you'll have about 240 working days a year. Multiply 15 patients a day by 240 workdays and you'll get 3,600 visits per year. Divide 3,600 visits by your estimated expenses for the year, and you'll come up with a figure of about $45 per visit.

For clarification, here is a partial listing of possible expenses you may incur: payroll (usually your largest expense), rent, telephone, medical and professional insurance, pension plan, professional licenses and dues, personnel expenses, equipment leases, postage, laundry, recruiting, clinical and office supplies, travel, maintenance, etc. Your income statement (see Chapter

13 and Appendix) will show your ongoing expenses. To better understand how expenses relate to guesstimated revenues in a start-up scenario, see the example of a pro-forma budget for a start-up clinic found in the Appendix.

When planning to contract with various managed care and other pre-paid insurance carriers, be sure that you will make more money with the carrier than it costs you to treat that patient. There are rarely any reasons to accept an offer to join any group that pays you equal or less than it costs you to do business. Margin or profit is realized only when you make more than you spend. In my calculation, the only reason to accept a patient whose insurance pays you less than your cost to provide the service is to woo or satisfy a potential referral source, who will be so pleased with your care that you will reap a future benefit from this one time or limited loss.

What's It All Cost, Alfie?

So, how do you know what to budget for? Money is spent in various ways in business. The main business expenditures you'll encounter are:

- ◆ **Capital Expenditures**—the physical assets you'll need, like furniture, computers, exercise equipment, and durable supplies
- ◆ **Start-up costs**—the costs related to getting the practice up and rolling in the marketplace. They include everything from brochure and prescription pad printing to installing equipment and buying soft goods.
- ◆ **Operating Losses**—losses that stem from the fact that you will not make money the day you generate the income. Briefly, since the majority of your patient bill is paid by third party payers, your turn-around time generally varies from two weeks to two years (not optimal!). Calculating how much you're in the loss column per month is important because you have to have the cash to cover these losses.
- ◆ **Fixed Costs**—expenditures that don't vary with the number of patients you see each month. They include rent, fixed salaries, and the like.

◆ **Variable Costs**—expenses that do vary with the volume of patients you see monthly. Examples of variable costs are soft goods, laundry services, and transcription costs.

Does This Venture Need to Cost Tons of Bucks?

You may think that to open a new practice, you would have to have more money than any bank or individual could possibly lend you. You will be surprised to learn that practices that open every day begin with significantly less than you can imagine. What's it all cost? The simple answer is that it all depends on:

◆ **What is the venture?**
◆ **How much office space do you need?**
◆ **What equipment will be purchased or leased?**
◆ **How much equipment do you need/want?**
◆ **What type and extent of furniture will be purchased?**
◆ **How many leasehold improvements are needed?**

In order to create a realistic start-up budget, your goal should always be to get into the black as fast as you can. In business jargon, we call that the *break-even point* (see next section). That means that you want to be familiar with and in control of your start-up costs, figure out your operating losses, and have a safety net in place for the months that your losses may exceed your cash collections. Your accountant will help you with these calculations and guesstimates. Your business plan will help you with crunching the necessary numbers to see when you expect to be in the black. Refer to the start-up pro-forma budget in the Appendix for revenue and expense line items to help you put your own budget in place.

Break Dancin' When You Break Even

Do you really want to know how much you'll need to budget to start your business? The break-even (BE) point is a good estimate to consider when calculating how many *shekels* you'll need. The BE point shows when your sales revenue (how much money you bring in) equals your total expenses (how much money you're paying out in expenses and salaries). The BE analysis is a mathematical formula. Don't be nervous about seeing numbers and graphs. We'll go one step at a time, starting with how the BE formula is developed, beginning with the cost-volume-profit (CVP) analysis.

The CVP analysis is the study of the effects of changes in costs and volume on a company's profits. CVP analysis is important in profit planning and also in setting your fee schedule (your prices), determining your best payer mix, and making the maximum use of your staff. CVP analysis involves a consideration of the interrelationships among your patient volume (sales volume), your fees, your cost to treat each patient (cost per unit), your total fixed costs, and your sales mix.

CVP analysis assumptions:

1. The behavior of your costs and revenues is linear.
2. All costs are classified as either variable or fixed.
3. Changes in activity are the only factors that affect costs.

The contribution margin (CM) is the amount of revenue remaining after subtracting the variable cost to provide the patient care treatment. The CM is mathematically defined as:

CM = Price per patient visit − Costs per patient visit

CM per visit indicates that for every patient visit, your business will have the CM to cover the fixed cost per visit (rent, salaries, etc.) and contribute to income (also called your *profit* or your *margin*).

Break-even analysis is the level of activity at which the total revenues equal total costs (both fixed costs and variable costs). At that specific volume of patient visits (sales), the business will realize no income and suffer no loss. The BE point can be expressed in either sales dollars (fees collected) or sales units (number of patient visits). Mathematically, it looks like this:

BE Sales = Variable Costs + Fixed Costs

Knowledge of the BE point is very useful to you in deciding whether to recruit more staff, buy more equipment, change your payer mix, or enter a new market.

A great way to derive the BE point is to prepare a BE graph. Since the graph also shows costs, volume of sales (number of patient visits), and profits, it is also referred to as the CVP graph. See the method of calculating the BE point and how to draw the graph in the Appendix.

It Costs Money to Make Money

OK, so you have a great location, a marketable niche, and referral sources lined up. You have calculated that you have a capital requirement of $50,000 to $100,000 to open this dream practice. Let's say you don't have a rich Aunt Ethel or Cousin Sadie who is dying to bankroll your new venture (or that you are not even in their respective wills). Now what?

Dig into Your Own Pockets, Pal

You may think that you have a well full of options to get money to start up your practice, including venture capitalists, banks, and other lending institutions. In fact, *Inc. Magazine*'s August 2003 issue reports that the leading sources of seed capital (start-up money) remain the so-called four Fs: founders, family, friends, and foolhardy investors. Seventy-nine percent of CEOs in Fortune 500 companies used personal savings to start up their ventures, 16% tapped family members' pocketbooks, 14% had a partner's cash, 10% used personal credit card lines, and 7% sought bank loans. According to an article in the September 2003 *MIT Enterprise Forum* newsletter, entrepreneurs tend to use personal savings, credit cards, personal credit lines, loans against their 401K, second mortgages, and seeking funds from trusted customers, relatives, and friends to finance their businesses. The bottom line is that the very high majority of practice starters finance their venture with their own personal resources with investments and/or loans from family, friends, and partners. The fact is, unless you are contemplating opening a mega-center with millions of dollars of equipment and services, a full service general orthopedic practice costs you less than $100,000 to start. Many may be able to open for much less. It all depends on the level and quantity of what you plan to buy for the practice and where you choose to locate it.

What About Banks Lending You Money?

The Small Business Administration (SBA), small business investment companies, and venture capitalists are not a primary resource for start-up capital for you. Why? Because they are looking for significant collateral and a quick, high return on their investment. Our business venture will hopefully be profitable, but the return on investment is slower than these groups want. In any event, if you have not been successful in generating start-up capital from your own pocket, Aunt Ethel's, or someone else's, your choice is narrowed to seeking funds from a bank. Understand that banks are in the business of lending money. The majority of their profits come from the interest they make on loans. They, of course, charge you more to "use" their money than they paid someone else (the depositors) to get it. The only catch here is that unless you have collateral to cover 100% of the loan, banks shy away from extending such a loan. Your collateral could include your home, your investments, and other assets you may own. Banks prefer to finance an existing, thriving business with a track record. If you have significant collateral, you may look to other lenders in the market, including the SBA, small business investment companies, venture capitalists, and minority funding organizations. Be prepared to complete volumes of paperwork, jump through hoops, and find your way out of red tape. The SBA's website, *www.sba.gov*, is your best resource for financing parameters and options. All told, in addition to your own money bags, your relatives and friends are your best bet to raise the necessary capital for your venture. Seems like everyone else does it. You can too!

What's the Equipment Cost? Can You Afford More? Can You Negotiate a Deal?

Nowadays, it's a breeze to find out ballpark prices. Search the Internet and compare prices with your local vendors. Set your browser to "physical therapy equipment" and you'll see hundreds of hits including such popular sites as *www.thesaundersgroup.com* and *www.therapyzone.com*. Locate your local vendors in the Yellow Pages. Meet with the local representative/salesman and shop prices with him, but know your prices ahead of time so you can negotiate with him or her. The sales representative will almost always negotiate better prices for more volume purchased.

 Never take the salesperson's initially offered price. Always counter the offer and request free shipping or other incentives.

For larger pieces of exercise equipment like a Kin-Com™ or Cybex™ isokinetic piece, I would suggest buying used. Most used equipment comes with a 90-day warranty or more, and many of the used treadmills and bikes come from fitness centers and spas that have closed down. The liquidated equipment is remanufactured and tuned up. The used equipment I have purchased over the years has served me well. For specifics on how the equipment is remanufactured and shined up, see the Megafitness link *http://www.megafitness.net/Remanufacturing-process.htm*. After reviewing this process and recognizing the much-reduced prices, you may never buy new again.

 Call local hospitals and rehabilitation centers. You'll be shocked to learn that if they have pieces of large equipment, they rarely use them. Be bold! Ask if they'd like to move out a large piece of their unused equipment to free up their tight space.

Recently I bought a Cybex isokinetic assessment and exercise device (Cybex NORM) that retailed new in 1998 for $60,000. I got it for a song—$6,000, from a local medical group that never used the device and felt it took up too much space. I use the equipment 10 times a day and laugh each time I put a patient on it.

There are websites dedicated to selling and servicing used, well maintained equipment, including *www.megafitness.com* and *www.rehabworld.com*. Another site that lists and sells used modality and exercise equipment is *www.medneeds.com*.

 Your web browser will direct you to hundreds more remanufactured equipment companies, but **buyer beware**! Check each seller's record with the Better Business Bureau (*www.bbbonline.org*) before you fork over your credit card number to the salesman. Don't say I didn't warn you.

When I decided to add a new treadmill and narrowed my choice to two online used equipment sellers, I checked with the Better Business Bureau online. One was a reputable company, while the other had multiple complaints lodged against it. The choice then was simple. When buying larger pieces of equipment, remember that shipping is expensive and buying from closer sources is always more cost effective.

From the previous section, you can easily imagine that a 500-square-foot space with "must have" furnishings only would be much less costly than a 3,000-square-foot state-of-the-art-equipped facility with top of the line computers, treatment modalities, and exercise devices. It's hard to imagine, but would you believe that opening a decent sized, 1,500-square-foot, well-appointed facility with some new and some used equipment and furniture could cost less than $50,000? Check out the math in the Appendix and see how it's done!

Without including operational costs like salaries, gas and electric, or maintenance fees, the total start-up outlay for our sample clinic shown in the Appendix is less than $50,000 for month number one. Obviously this is oversimplifying things a bit, but it is meant to illustrate that opening the doors of a generous-sized clinic with a fair amount of equipment meant to accommodate a 15 to 20 patient-a-day caseload can cost less than $50,000 to open. Granted, you have to produce patients and aggressively collect fees to generate your salary on top of paying back these expenses quickly so as not to continue a downhill spiral of expenses overwhelmingly outweighing income.

In your business plan (see Chapter 5 for details), you will create a budget to numerically demonstrate how much money you will actually require to start up and move your business forward. It should also show when you plan to begin taking a salary, the BE point, and when you will realize a profit. Start-up businesses typically run into trouble when the owners do not plan their steps of action and, as such, set themselves up for potential failure. I cannot emphasize enough the importance of proper planning during each and every step of the way.

Who Sells the Cheapest Furniture?

If you have the cash and want a totally new palace, don't read this section. In my humble opinion, buying shiny, new file cabinets to house shelves full of multi-colored patient charts that hide almost every inch of shelf space is ridiculous. File cabinets are made sturdy to hold the weight of the multitude of charts and will develop dings and scratches shortly after they are bought new. So why bother? Many large cities have used office furniture dealers who buy out inventories from major corporations when they go out of business. You will find great deals there by mixing and matching fabrics, designs, and sizes, and you should always negotiate volume discounts (one chair is $45, so how much for ten chairs?) or free or discounted delivery costs.

 Recently, I walked into a store called Office Furniture Liquidators and bought two brand name lateral file cabinets that cost $690 new (I checked the new price on the Internet), both for only $150. Sure they had a few dents, but who would see them? They threw in free delivery and set up. Places like this frequently add inventory, so going in once a week or so will give you different options and possibilities. You can generally match sizes and styles of cabinets, desks, and chairs since they usually buy out a company's total lot all at once.

If you insist on buying new (and are reading this section even though I told you not to), Staples® and Office Depot® offer relatively cheap prices and free delivery on new office furniture and filing systems. Generally, both stores offer free delivery on any order more than $50. For schlepping furniture, that's an incredible deal. If I still have not convinced you to buy used or at a discount and you want to buy retail, there are several office furniture showrooms in most cities, listed in the Yellow Pages, who have their wares in place so you can see how they look in groups and what fabric matches which desk laminate color.

 When choosing chairs and desks, new or used, buy quality. In your waiting room you may have Mrs. Portly who weighs 295 pounds and just had a hip replacement plopping down on your chair. It better support her well or you may have a new suit—

not a three-piece pinstripe banker's gray suit either, but a lawsuit instead!

Remember our professional mission to encourage correct body mechanics. Buy functional and biomechanically correct and comfortable chairs and desks for you, your staff, and your patients. Pay attention to workstation ergonomics so that your staff does not end up out of work on worker's comp charges.

I know the price of success: dedication, hard work, and an unremitting devotion to the things you want to see happen.

—*Frank Lloyd Wright*

CHAPTER 4

You Can Bank on It!

What? I Have to Pay to Keep My Money in the Bank?

If you have only had a private, personal account in a bank where they woo you in any way possible to keep your money with them, you will be as surprised as I was to learn that banks make good money on business accounts. It's hard to believe, but every time you use your bank, whether to deposit money, move money, withdraw money, or pay bills via the bank, it will cost you. Most banks offer rate sheets that fully disclose their fees for commercial accounts. Some offer incentives to draw you to their banks, like free "for deposit only" rubber stamps or free checks for new business customers even though their fees may be the same or more than other local banks. Recently, along with federally insured commercial banks, local credit unions have been allowed to enroll private businesses as customers, and they have been offering incentives like no-fee checking, no-fee deposits, or free online banking for business customers.

Shop Till You Drop (Drop Your Money in That Account, That Is)

A good businessman will shop the banks and credit unions to find the best rates while keeping in mind convenience and location of the bank. A bank with minimal to no monthly fees located 36 miles from your practice or home is no bargain compared to a banking institution that charges acceptable fees and has branches next door to your office and a block from your home. Once you pick your bank, you'll deposit some of the money Aunt Ethel loaned you to start your dream business.

Teller, Teller, Tell Me Do: What Information Does My Bank Need?

The bank officer will need your name, business address, phone number, tax ID number, and will ask for a PIN to keep your information confidential and available only to you. You'll pick out a checkbook style and color. I always recommend checkbooks with attached stubs because they are easier to maintain when it comes to the month-end balancing act. The bank clerk will give you some blank checks to use until your custom order arrives. Estimate that your custom order will arrive within two weeks by courier.

Speaking of checks, don't forget about payroll checks. Your employees surely won't! There are two ways to do payroll: in-house or outsourcing. If you outsource it, contact companies such as ADP (*www.adp.com*) or Paychex (*www.paychex.com*). There are local companies as well. Your accountant may know of some, or you can ask other trusted business owners you know.

If you plan on doing your own payroll in-house like I do with software such as Quickpay (*www.quicken.com*), you'll need to order payroll checks with voucher stubs. There are several types and styles of payroll checks with voucher stubs on the side of the check or under the actual check. Your check style choice is determined by the payroll software you use. I order my checks from Compuchecks (*www.compuchecks.com*) and find them to be very reliable and timely. They print and ship the order within five days. "Rush same day" processing and shipping is available at a minimal extra cost. I order 300 voucher checks printed with my company name, address, and logo, and they mail the order directly to me for less than $40, including shipping. Many other discount check printing companies can be found to work with your individual accounting, bookkeeping, or payroll software. Set your web browser to "discount computer checks" and watch how many hits you get!

Check, Please!

Most businesses operate only with a checking account, funneling necessary funds in and out for payroll and liability expenses (accounts payable bills and taxes to be paid). Some practitioners also avail themselves of investment vehicles in their banks to generate interest while their money sits in the bank. This is usually recommended only if you are fortunate enough to generate enough money that is not immediately needed to pay your employees or other debts. Generally, the owners (called principals) of the business usually transfer extra monies into other investment accounts (or into their own pocket as bonuses) and maintain only a checking account.

The secret of joy in work is contained in one word—excellence. To know how to do something well is to enjoy it.

—*Pearl Buck*

CHAPTER 5

Plan to Win

What's a Mission Statement and Do I Need One?

Who are you and what makes you and your upcoming practice different, sharper, or better than Joe's next door? You're on a mission, and that mission is to create a written definition of your practice's purpose. It is a clear statement of who and what you are. It should identify you and your practice to others, including your famous four bosses: your patients (both present and future), your referring practitioners (your daily bread), your staff (your new extended family), and your payers (the guys paying your way).

The mission statement is brief and catchy. It should be easy to remember and always on the tip of your and your staff's tongues.

Examples of mission statements include:

◆ **Nordstrom:** "We exceed customers' expectations."
◆ **Disney:** "To make people happy."
◆ **Boeing:** "To push the leading edge of aviation, taking on huge challenges doing what others cannot do."
◆ **Mary Kay:** "To give unlimited opportunity to women."

When composing your mission statement, use creativity after reviewing others' successful statements. DO NOT copy someone else's mission statement that is copyrighted or is clearly recognizable as created by another organization. Like Nordstrom, if customer satisfaction is paramount to your practice, say so. If you want to keep your referral sources happy, think like Disney. In any event, your mission statement creation is truly a mission—to clearly and cleverly describe your practice in a brief, easy-to-recall thought. Now, once you have your mission statement in mind, you have to get it to stick in everyone else's mind as well. Post the mission statement on your door, clinic wall, in your business plan, and on the cover of your employee manual. Post it EVERYWHERE, even perhaps in the restrooms! Esterson & Associates' mission statement is based on Nordstrom's idea: *"We will exceed your expectations in our attention to your needs and outstanding level of care."*

I've Got 20/20: Do I Still Need a Vision?

Yes, you should create a vision for your practice. While the mission statement summarizes the what, how, and why of an organization's work, a vision statement presents a creative image of what success will look like. The company's vision is the bar you want your staff to visualize as they pole-vault over the competition. How do you come up with a vision? Include your staff in a brainstorming session to develop ideas. Use a powerful image that describes a goal for your practice. Martin Luther King, Jr. said, "I have a dream," and what followed was a vision that changed our nation forever. Often metaphors are used to accent the statement and enhance self-visualization of the words. The vision becomes reachable, easily understood by all, appropriate, and consistent with the business direction, values, and morals. Briefly, it should inspire anyone who reads it, especially your staff, to achieve the practice's mission and vision. Here are a few examples of vision statements:

- ◆ **Our organization is like ... a mariachi band—all playing the same music together, or like a train—pulling important cargo and laying the track as we go (from *http://www. allianceonline.org/search/searchframe.cfm*).**
- ◆ **The Great American Forest, since our nation's founding, has provided the resources to build our homes, our schools, our churches—it has provided the inspiration for our philosophers, our poets, our artists. Working together we can continue to improve, enhance, and protect this great natural resource to help ensure that we have healthy forests with clean water, clean air, abundant wildlife, wilderness,**

and working forests in harmony with the needs of all
Americans and for the generations yet to come (from
http://www.yale.edu/forest_congress/vision.html).

◆ Our vision is to be a world-class organization—one that
becomes a benchmark for other organizations, so they
can copy what we do and get it right in about five years,
by which time we will be light years ahead of them (from
http://www.betterworkplacenow.com/qanda1.html).

What's a Business Plan? Should I Plan on Writing One?

Yes, you definitely need a business plan for several reasons.
First, it forces you to put down on paper exactly what you are
planning to do with your cash, your time, your efforts, and your
location, down to the most minute detail. Why do you need it?
You need to use the business plan as your map and compass to
give direction to your start-up practice. If you require financing
(called "capital" in the business world), banks and other lending institutions, both private and public, demand to know why
in the world you need tens or hundreds of thousands of *shekels*
to open the practice of your dreams. The business plan gives
these executives or rich cousins the whole story.

In short, business gurus define the business plan as a formal,
written document approximately 50 pages long, which states
the purposes, methods, and goals of your business venture and
describes in detail how you plan on attaining those goals. It is
ideally written before a practice opens its doors because it acts
as a feasibility test. If you do a good job of researching your
business, making your business decisions, and doing your financial projections, then you can have a good idea ahead of time
whether or not your business will work. The business plan is not
meant to be a final, unchangeable document. Rather, it is flexible and open to change as time unfolds. Many professionals
use it to gauge their financial performance, comparing actual
performance with initial projections. When creating your business plan, you'll need a *pro-forma* balance sheet for the next
two years. Pro-forma means that you are using projections
instead of actual figures to estimate your future sales (number
of patient visits) and growth. To get a better picture of a pro-

forma layout, see my sample pro-forma budget in the Appendix. You will learn more about balance sheets and other accounting statements in Chapter 13. The size of the plan is not as important as its accuracy and *glitz* (how much you make your intended venture shine and appear like a real winner). Knock the reader's socks off. Make it so convincingly good that he or she wants to read each page fully. Everyone likes clear and understandable charts and outlines. Stay simple and concise. Spend time and good money on creating and collating a professional looking document. Beware of grammar and spelling errors; they can ruin your otherwise wonderful plan. Use your computer software, like MS Word® and Excel®, to write the document. Places like Kinko's© and Sir Speedy© can dress up your business plan with glossy covers and colorful charts.

The following is a sample business plan table of contents and a description of each section:

Part I: The Practice
    a. The mission and vision statements
    b. Summary of the practice
    c. Legal description of the practice
    d. The competition and your edge over them

Part II: The Management Team
Describe the people involved and don't be modest. Brag about as much as you can to accurately convince the investor that you deserve their money. Who better than you can boast about your abilities, skills, and drive to succeed?

Part III. The Marketing Plan
Describe the industry (physical therapy in a global way), your competition, your potential customers (referring practitioners and patients), and how you'll get them in your door and into your clutches.
    a. The industry—who are the leaders, how competitive is the market, and who else does what you do?
    b. The potential customers
    c. The location
    d. Advertising—How? When? How much? To whom?

Part IV. The Management Plan

Who is on the team? How much are they paid? What are the benefits and fringe incentives? Describe the employee manual. What are the future financial opportunities on the horizon?

Part V. Risks

Identify and explain the risks of the practice and how you plan to surmount them.

Part VI. The Financial Management Plan

Show realistically projections of the financial side of your dream. Use a pro-forma report in a spreadsheet format (i.e., MS Excel®). A sample of a pro-forma report is found in the Appendix.

The Small Business Administration (SBA), found at *http://www.sba.gov*, is an agency of the federal government that has extensive information on its website about all aspects of business development, management, and productivity.

There are a wide variety of books about writing clear and concise business plans that attract the eye of the reader. Try these two books I used to create my own business plan:

Arkebauer, J. B. (1995). The McGraw-Hill Guide to Writing a High-Impact Business Plan. New York: McGraw-Hill.
Berle, G., & Kirschner, P. (1997). The Instant Business Plan. Santa Maria: Puma Publishing.

 Now that you've finished your plan, keep it readily accessible. Many people use their original business plan to review their initial goals to see if they were met. You may use the plan as a springboard for future growth, and to reflect back on why you thought to even enter this venture in the first place. By the way, if you don't feel secure in knowing that you can write your own business plan, there are tons of canned plans on the market (for about $50–$100), as well as consulting groups that will be more than happy to take your money (to the tune of hundreds or thousands of dollars) and develop a glossy, professional display of your enterprise. For further ideas and tips, set your Internet browser to "business plans" and sit back and watch how many hits you'll get. Try the SBA's website, *www. sba.gov; www.bplans.com; www.businessplanarchive.org; www. morebusiness.com;* and *www.myownbusinessorg,* among others.

In this age of technology, there is really no excuse not to have an outstanding business plan whether you do it yourself, use a canned fill-in-the-blank software program, or outsource it. Lastly, have a colleague or friend review the plan for ease of reading and clarity. Let them mark it up and change what you feel is necessary.

Now That I've Got a Plan, What Next?

A sizeable chunk of your planning is now over. You've identified what it is you want to create and you've pinpointed the means by which you'll tackle it. Can you do it alone even if you are a sole proprietor? Don't even think of it. You need a team of experts and advisors that at least includes an accountant and an attorney to guide and advise you through your beginning steps in realizing your dream practice.

Destiny is not a matter of chance; it is a matter of choice. It is not a thing to be waited for, it is a thing to be achieved.

—*William Jennings Bryan*

CHAPTER **6**

The Dream Team

Who's with Me?

Business is so involved that you need more advice than your
own mother-in-law gives you for free. The best way to get this
advice is to have a group of professionals and perhaps colleagues or mentors that work with you to guide you on the most
functional and realistic trail. Call it your foundation team.
What will the dream team offer? They'll discuss and help you
understand and decide on the following:

- ◆ **What legal structure do I want or need for my practice?**
- ◆ **What tax ramification issues will I encounter in choosing the legal structure?**
- ◆ **What are my responsibilities as a business owner?**
- ◆ **What kind of cash do I really need to open my practice?**
- ◆ **What size suite do I need to lease?**
- ◆ **What is the best geographic location for my practice?**
- ◆ **What are my marketing needs?**
- ◆ **What are my management needs?**
- ◆ **What formal documents must I obtain before opening my doors?**
- ◆ **What is necessary for compliance with federal, state, and local regulations and laws?**

How Do I Choose an Attorney and What Should I Expect?

In the beginning, the attorney's function is to:

- ◆ **Advise you on the best legal organization for your practice.**
- ◆ **Prepare the necessary documents for your practice.**

♦ **Review leases and other contracts.**
♦ **Help you comply with federal, state, and local regulations and laws.**
♦ **Represent your interests in legal actions.**

Like healthcare professionals, attorneys specialize in different aspects of the law: tax, litigation, corporate, real estate, business mergers, etc. Look for a corporate attorney with experience in tax law.

Choose your attorney carefully because he or she will be your partner in your practice for all intents and purposes. He or she will advise you on matters that most likely you have little to no experience with so that you can make an informed decision. Ask friends, colleagues, mentors, and relatives whom they recommend. Interview the candidates and be sure that you share similar mindsets about business ethics, customer service, and trust. Compatibility is crucial as this will hopefully be a long-term relationship.

As one who is starting up a new practice, feel free to ask for flexible, easy terms and fees, and expect consideration and attention despite your current small size. Assess the attorney's attitude toward you when you call and pay attention to how staff treat you. Check if he or she has flexible hours in case you wish to meet in the evenings or on weekends. In short—choose a firm with a solid reputation, one that can grow with you, and one with other specialties so that when you expand, the firm will have the necessary advisors for you.

One, Two, Three: See, I Can Count. So, Why an Accountant?

You need an accountant to maintain your overall financial fitness and to do the following:

♦ **Set up your books and instruct you on what taxes you'll need to pay and when to pay them.**

◆ **Establish systems to track and maintain your income, out-flows (payments out), and tax liabilities.**

◆ **Advise you on areas such as accounts payable and receivable.**

Choose your accountant the same way you choose your other dream team members—by recommendations from others. He or she should have a similar work ethic as you and a compatible business style.

Even before you open your doors, your accountant will be on your payroll. According to your choice and needs, he or she may be involved more or less in the everyday running of your practice, like writing your checks and balancing your checkbook, or may act only as an advisor at month end or quarter end to run your financials.

Like your attorney, find an accountant who can grow with you and is approachable and readily available when you need him or her. We will discuss tax liabilities and other accounting code words in a later chapter.

I'm Already Broke, So Why an Insurance Broker?

Before you open your doors, you will need malpractice insurance, property and casualty insurance, unemployment insurance, worker's compensation insurance, medical insurance, and maybe others. Who has time to shop the multitude of carriers to find the most cost-effective premiums? You could call one of hundreds of insurance agents found in the Yellow Pages under large corporations like State Farm or Nationwide. On the other hand, I have always been partial to independent brokers because I see them as business owners like me, trying to increase their clientele.

Find a reputable independent broker who looks out for you and keeps you abreast of all changes in your coverage. Good brokers will call and offer to switch you to a better plan at lower premium rates. Interview all potential candidates for your business like you did for your accountant and lawyer. Always ask for references and look for personality traits with which you feel comfortable. Feel free to shop around for the best premium package.

Bringing in the Dough: Knead a Billing Consultant?

The complexities of insurance billing are so overwhelming nowadays that even the most experienced practitioners are toying with outsourcing their billings. Most large metropolitan areas have a large payer mix, including commercial carriers (such as Blue Cross), preferred provider organizations (such as Aetna), managed care groups (such as Kaiser-Permanente), auto insurers (such as Geico), and worker's compensation carriers (such as Injured Worker's Insurance Fund and Kemper).

Having adequate staff and the computer software to electronically bill the carriers and then follow up on their slow payment is a daunting task, not even considering the inside cost of it. Many practitioners begin by hiring an experienced billing person. In addition to this expense, you will pay top dollar for your billing software program and an electronic billing intermediary. Software itself costs in the thousands of dollars and may also have a yearly license fee. When you add another billing clerk and need to network your hardware system, you may incur another fee for adding a module to allow multiple-screen-viewing of the same data. The advantage of keeping your billing in-house is that you can monitor and supervise all your billings on site. Everything will be under your proverbial nose.

Others, who prefer to maintain the hair left on their heads, choose another possibility—outsourcing. Find a billing group who can collate, bill, collect, post, and report on all aspects of your billing for you. This is a decent system that many prefer. The outsourced company has an incentive to collect the most money possible because you pay it a percentage of the return.

On a personal note, I have been quite successful outsourcing my billing. It saves me office space, supervisory aggravation, the cost of securing and maintaining a billing system, and the payroll expense of supporting a billing/collection staff. Despite the fact that the billing is not under my direct supervision, I can watch the process on my computer screen in addition to scrutinizing monthly reports. The going rate for outsourcing such a deal is between 6 and 10%. As with the other consultants, you can never lose by asking the billers to work with you to begin with a low percentage and gradually increase to an agreed upon figure as the business grows. The worst they can say is no.

When toying with outsourcing versus doing your own billing, consider this: to bill in-house, you'll need computer hardware, a hardware service contract, billing software, ongoing software support and upgrades (a continual expense), and, of course, dedicated, aggressive, experienced, and financially savvy personnel to collect your money. Ignoring the initial outlay of cash for hardware (say, a few thousand dollars), your major cost is personnel. Two experienced insurance clerks may run you $75,000 a year or more. To pay out that sum to an outsource company charging a commission of say 7%, you'd need to collect a bit more than $1,000,000. Avoiding the aggravation, frustration, and disgust when the billing hardware breaks down, the software locks up, the staff call in sick, security and privacy breaches ring the Health Insurance Portability and Accountability Act bell, and the toll-free software support phone line is busy are other reasons to consider outsourcing your billing.

 If you do choose to do the billing yourself, there are multitudes of software billing programs and some include practice management and scheduling modules. I have been impressed with TherapySoft (*http://www.therapysoftware.com*) and Turbo PT by Global Support Systems (*http://www.gssinc.com*), among others. It is best to visit other practices on the other side of town (those who are not your competition) to investigate their software experiences and preferences, likes and dislikes.

My recommendation would be to hire an experienced billing person before your doors open to help choose a software billing program that he or she is either already familiar with or impressed with. I have had a very good experience with a local software engineer's product that many area medical and physical therapy groups use. The advantage is that he is close by and available for consultation should I hit a curve in the road. The disadvantage is that he is a small player in a big market, so his system may not meet everyone's global needs.

Your vision will become clear only when you look inside your heart. Who looks outside, dreams. Who looks inside, awakens.

—*Carl Jung*

CHAPTER 7

Setting Up Shop

Where on This Green Earth Do I Locate This Venture?

Location, location, location are the three most commonly heard words when asking why a given business prospers. In physical therapy, locating next to a group of orthopedic surgeons who think you have the best hands in the world seems likely to be a gold mine for you. On the other hand, locating your venture between a used car lot and the city landfill with no potential referring practitioners or medical facilities nearby seems fruitless. Here's my story and the lessons I learned about the importance of location.

When I first ventured out on my own, I chose to get a free map from AAA, tack it to my wall, open the local Yellow Pages, and put a colorful pushpin at every spot there was a Yellow Pages listing of a private physical therapy practice or hospital outpatient clinic in the metropolitan area. After that I stood back, gazed at the map full of pushpins and noticed that there was not a practice to be found along the west side corridor of the county. A pre-Internet basic demographic investigation with the county Chamber of Commerce (brochures, lists of population demographics, neighborhoods, maps) enlightened me of the limited light industry and significant number of federal agency facilities in the area. Without hesitation I realized that I would locate my castle there and immediately began what I felt at the time was appropriate planning.

Since I had limited previous business experience, less than a solid business plan, or this excellent book in hand when I opened my first practice in 1985, I admit that my initial choice for my clinic location was less than optimal. I could not believe that after doing what I felt was decent planning, opening my doors, waiting for that first fortunate soul to enter who would benefit from my care, and only getting a trickle of patients after weeks of being open for business, I had made any business blunders. With 20–20 retrospective vision, I now know that the reason was that there were no physicians or other potential referral sources in the vicinity. Who in their right mind would open in a place devoid of referring practitioners?

Now what? Being an entrepreneur, I had to regroup and rethink the scenario. How could I still make this a winning situation? It was at that moment that I discovered the meaning of a "niche practice."

Real Therapists Don't Open **Niche** Practices

Well this therapist surely did! After coming to the cold realization that I had fallen into a hole, the entrepreneurial spirit burned within me! How was I going to generate business in a market without referral sources in close proximity? My demographic research before opening in this location showed me that I had industry and federal agencies employing over 40,000 people within a two-mile radius. So my next step was figuring out which orthopedists were seeing this population. Where were these employees getting their primary care? To what extent is managed care involved in patient referrals? Read on.

What's Your Pleasure? General, Specialized, or Niche?

Bottom Line: You need people to come in your door and seek your care. What population are you looking for? Do you want to see only adult patients with musculoskeletal and neuromuscular problems? That is usually called a general practice. How about only sports injuries or just kids? That's called a specialized practice. Another type of practice is called a niche practice. A niche can be a slot, place, or function, an untapped area perhaps. In my situation, I realized that I had no close referral sources but discovered that a large government agency that employs about 30,000 people is a mile from my new facility. Shouldn't I have known this before? Sure, I should have, but I naively counted on establishing a physical presence where others hadn't yet discovered instead of choosing a location based upon the population-need, referral potential, convenience factors, and physical space quality.

 Even if people live 25 miles from my office, they work around the corner. I needed to market myself to practitioners far from the clinic, advertising that I can see their patients who live or work in the west corridor of the county, and that I offer early morning and late evening hours for the convenience of the working patient. I sent letters saying, "I am your Western County choice physical therapist" to as many primary care practitioners and orthopedists as I could find in the Yellow Pages. I highlighted my location and extensive hours for the convenience of the working patient, along with my contact numbers. I hand wrote the word "Confidential" on the envelope so I would be sure that the physician himself opened it. I can't tell you what a great niche-marketing trick that was. We were so busy in such a short time that we needed to double, then triple our staff in a matter of six months. Such rapid success stories may be rare, but with planning and good forethought, compared to 20/20 hindsight, you can also make it happen virtually anywhere in town!

Do I Need a License to Open This Business?

It goes without saying that you, of course, DO need a state license to practice physical therapy in any capacity. Your license must be displayed in a conspicuous place in full view of your customers. In addition, some states require any and all business owners to obtain a business license of some sort. Some states only require retail establishments to obtain a business license. Service industries like physical therapy that do not specifically sell tangible, taxable items do not require a business license. Some insurance carriers require physical therapists to hold a "letter of good standing." This is to apparently certify that you are worthy to contract with and that you have not amassed stacks of unpaid parking tickets in the community.

Further, in order to become a Medicare provider in Maryland, you must obtain a "letter of good standing" from the state's Department of Assessments and Taxation. How do you get such a letter? Believe it or not, you simply mail or fax a letter indicating that you are the principal (owner) of a business and are applying for a letter of good standing. The clerk researches whether you are a convicted felon and have been cleared of those charges, or have paid the outstanding parking tickets. Then they will send you a very official looking document, sporting a gold seal and all, stating that you are a business in good standing in the State of Maryland after, of course, you mail in a check for $12.

Space Out!

Office configurations vary greatly, but they all at least have the following five areas:

- ◆ **Waiting Room**   ◆ **Gym Area**
- ◆ **Receptionist Area**   ◆ **Offices**
- ◆ **Patient Treatment Rooms**

How Do You Know What You Want or Need?

Well, one way is to visit a number of existing practices in your area and scribble down a list of what you love about an office's layout and what you feel are impediments to patient "flow." Restrooms may be internal to the suite, or a shared restroom may be in the hallway of a multi-use building suite. For convenience sake, inside facilities are preferred. When planning bathrooms and sinks, be sure that you are in compliance with the Americans with Disabilities Act of 1990 (ADA). To read the statute in full *legalese*, log onto *http://www.eeoc.gov/ laws/ ada.html*. For complete information on technical assistance and design standards, set your Internet browser to *http:// www.usdoj.gov/crt/ada/adahom1.htm*.

You may want to do your own laundering of towels and pillowcases. In that case, you'll need space and a hookup for a washer-dryer set. You'll need some cabinets and closets for towels and other assorted equipment and supplies. By the way, Medicare rules specify that clean towels are to be in a closed cabinet. Warehouse dealers like Home Depot® and Lowe's® offer great prices on standard cabinets and work countertops.

One helpful tip regarding planning for electrical outlets is to place an outlet 48″ above the floor in your treatment rooms. That way you'll easily be able to move your ultrasound unit or electrical stimulation machine without repetitively bending over to reach a floor plug in each exam room. Consider the need for ground fault outlets in areas where there is water, like in a whirlpool room. Ground fault outlets have built-in breakers that shut down when exposed to water, thereby avoiding shock to the operator of the equipment or the patient.

Wait Just a Minute!

Do you need a larger waiting room because your potential patients will bring their Aunt Gussie and Cousin Sue with her 12 children? If not, save the few square feet for a larger business office. Office suites are based on square footage. You may envision a small, cozy office with two treatment tables, free weights, some Theraband®, and an exercise bike. To calculate such a space requirement, measure out the space of the actual equipment, add one third more space for patient walk-through, sprinkle in some area for a few waiting room chairs, including double the chair area space for walk-through and sufficient space for your mother-in-law who will be your receptionist, and add an extra room for towels and a sink. Voila! You have just calculated your dream suite.

 A more exact idea is to buy an inexpensive house-space-planning software program available at stores like CompUSA® and Best Buy®. Plugging in the floor square footage footprint area of your equipment, desk, and other furniture, the program then prints out a clear diagram in either a two or three-dimensional format. Handing an organized floor plan like this to your landlord will win you a friend for life.

 I have had recent requests from workmen's comp insurance carriers asking me the square footage of my clinic, to list the exercise equipment and modalities I own and employ in the clinic, and if I have a therapeutic pool. This specific carrier requires its credentialed providers to have at least a 1,500 square foot clinic and 500 square foot gym area. This carrier is clearly making a statement that it wants a therapeutic environment for its injured worker and not a modality-only approach. This may be the beginning of third party carriers directing their customers to clinics of given sizes and equipment types. Perhaps these carriers want to begin referring to what they will determine are clinics of excellence. Stay tuned and informed for more on that topic.

Now I'm Really **Spacing Out**: Do I Need a Space Planner?

Now that I know where I want to set up shop, I have to figure out what I'll need for office space. Your best bet is to begin with a "shell" or an empty space that can be subdivided according to your own design. In designing your office, consider all present and anticipated future needs. If you will require water, include a sink in your plan. If you expect to enlarge your practice one day, include treatment areas that you may not even occupy initially. If you plan to automate and computerize the office, be sure to have the contractor include dedicated lines for a fax or broadband communication. One thing you can't have too much of is closet and storage space. Make sure you give yourself plenty of room to store treatment and office supplies, books, financial records, archived patient charts, and the like.

Some people are blessed with a three-dimensional perspective when sketching out a design. Others are not. If you are in the "not" group, look for a space planner in the Yellow Pages under "Interior Design." The space planner will take your needs and ideas and draw up designs that will maximize your space and offer a proper flow for patients and staff. They also may have connections for obtaining office furniture and storage cabinets at bulk prices.

At a course I took with one of the physical therapist management gurus, Peter Kovacek, he advised calling local universities' and colleges' art and design educational programs and proposing a special project to a chosen student to design and lay out an office interior for you. That way, you get your cake and eat it too. You get the benefit of the student's design (and perhaps his or her advisor's input too) at a cost of zero or next to nothing.

When Is a Lease Not a **Leash?**

Your lease is the written, legal document between you or your corporation and the landlord. Most leases are voluminous and full of *legalese*, the language that only your attorney speaks. Leigh Gallagher, in her article *"The Lease You Can Do"* in the 1996 September/October issue of the *Philadelphia Enterpriser*, identified eight items your lease should always include to protect you and your practice:

1. **Flexibility**: The length of the lease should match the projected needs of the business.
2. **Cancellation rights**: Try to negotiate a mid-lease cancellation option for protection, should the business venture fail.
3. **Expansion options**: Make sure your space can grow with the business.
4. **Assignment and subletting options**: Be sure that the lease allows you to freely sublet whatever space you don't use, including the entire space if your business explodes and you have to move.
5. **Escalation provisions**: Terms and conditions outlined in business leases often allow for increases in building operational costs that can cause rent to skyrocket. Convince the landlord to document operating expenses for the past three years before signing the lease.
6. **Details about services furnished by the landlord**: Be sure that the lease clearly spells out how certain services will be provided (for example, what hours will the exterior lights be on, and is the heat turned off automatically after 5 P.M.).
7. **Nondisturbance provisions/subordination**: Negotiate "quiet enjoyment," that is, be sure that if the current landlord sells the building, the new landlord can't evict you if he finds a tenant willing to pay more than you do for your space.
8. **Terms of default**: Besides simply not paying your rent on time, there are a number of ways to default on your lease. There should always be a remedy to any breach in the agreement.

NEVER, I repeat **NEVER**, sign a lease without having your attorney approve it first. Landlords notoriously put all kinds of caveats and twists in the lease that favor them in the event of a catastrophe, like a flood from a broken pipe. You never want your lease to be a leash restraining you from doing what you intended to do in the office suite. My first lease had a line that said that in the event there was a dispute between the landlord and me that found its way to court, I would waive my right to a jury trial. That's ridiculous, but the landlord tried to slip it in anyway. My attorney, at the time, slashed his red pen through tens of lines of such foolishness and the landlord smiled and signed the document anyway. Don't ever think that the landlord is out to save you any money.

At Lease You Have a Beautiful Office Suite

How do you know what the going rate is for leasing office space in your chosen area? Simple—go to five or ten other buildings in the area and speak to the landlords there. Numbers quoted are in dollar amount per square foot per lease year. When a landlord says that a 1,500 square foot space rents for $14.95 a square foot, that means the space will cost you $22,425 per year; divided by 12 months this is $1868.75 a month. Glitzy, well-appointed suites in a highly visible location may cost you $25 to $50 a square foot compared to a privately owned modest medical building at $12.50 a square foot. Check if the square footage cost includes gas, electric, janitorial, and common area maintenance fees (costs of keeping the grounds, exterior lights, and hallways maintained) for your suite. Even though it is preferable for you as a tenant to have it all inclusive, most landlords don't want the headache of worrying about your interior space and would rather have you pay your own heat and electric bill, clean your own mess, and charge you out the kazoo for keeping their lot, grounds, and hallways maintained. If it is an all-inclusive lease, you pay the same fee every month and the landlord has to have the aggravation of paying differing amounts for each month's heat and electric bills and maintenance. Square footage may not be exact and may be termed a "rental unit" or "module" in the lease. This reference to your space protects the landlord when you decide to actually measure your suite length and width and come up with a few square feet less than what the landlord stated in the lease agreement. Be sure the lease contains reference to the hours you will be open so that parking lot lights will remain on in the evenings you are there. Do you need more handicapped parking spaces in front of your entrance? That too can be put into the lease. You can even negotiate that a given number of spots close to your suite's entrance will be reserved for your patients' parking. Is your rest room ADA approved? That should be on the drawings and in the lease.

Punch List or Forever Hold Your Piece!

The lease document often has addenda and appendices with office build-out drawings and a *punch list*. A punch list is a list of what mechanical fix-ups are needed before the office space is completed. When the landlord signs the lease document containing the punch list, it is a promise that even after he or she provides you, the tenant, with the office key, he or she is bound to add or fix items you have specified. These items may be as simple as repairing a doorknob or as complex as adding a doorway that was omitted from your original plans. Always go through the finished build-out with the landlord (called a "walk through") and note every item that needs attention. Turn every doorknob, flick every light switch on and off, flush every toilet, run every sink faucet, and check all the electric outlets to be sure they work. After the document is signed, you have no recourse and the landlord is off the hook.

 Be totally sure everything is on the build-out drawing before you sign the lease. If the landlord is paying for the build-out, as is often the case, if it's not on the drawing, the landlord won't be responsible to complete it. The rent escalation table is also in the lease. This table shows you what you are paying each year of the lease term. Most leases are for a minimum of three to five years with a 5% increase each year. Don't feel embarrassed to ask the landlord for a few months free rent when you first open. He's usually happy to have a stable, clean, honest tenant that will most likely be around for years to come. Always review the lease terms and have others look it over for accuracy. Once you sign on the dotted line, you're stuck with the contents of the lease.

It never hurts to ask for the sky. If the landlord is hungry enough, you'd be surprised at the perks he or she will offer just to have you as a tenant. The longer the term the landlord ropes you in as a tenant, the more freebies he or she is usually willing to throw in. I have always signed for terms no longer than five years. If you're more of a risk taker, you may want to agree to a 10-year term with more flexibility in terms and payment schedules.

The Technology You Can't Do Without

In our generation of automation, you must computerize your office in order to maintain patient data, prepare and process billing, and generate letters to referral sources. From a hardware perspective, you should buy computer equipment that is top of the line without spending on all the bells and whistles you'll never need. For example, local electronics retailers like Best Buy or CompUSA have weekly circulars in the newspapers hawking desktop computers. Any one of the systems listed would most likely be more than enough for your needs. Online and mail order companies like Dell® (*www.dell.com*), IBM® (*www.ibm.com*), and Gateway® (*www.gateway.com*) have outstanding buys, incentives, and deals on a regular basis. Shipping is often cheap or free. In fact, many therapists are still aligned with their universities and have accessibility to the school's computer educational deals. Don't miss out! Call your school and find out if you are eligible to purchase computers through them.

Virtually all universities work deals with the major computer hardware and software companies. The computer companies rely on volume sales to the university and, in turn, offer the faculty, staff, and student body percentages off hardware and peripherals (various network cards, Ethernet wireless cards, printers, cables, etc.). Through my university affiliation, first as a student and now as a faculty member, I "built" my own computer to my specifications for 10% less than the prices in discount stores like Best Buy and CompUSA. I also got free shipping, a further discount for purchasing two computer systems, and a 50% off mail-in rebate for a router to network the two systems together. If you are not a computernik, ask friends, colleagues, or teachers who are computer-savvy to help you design and "build" a system that will work best for you. Each computer company's website affiliated with your university has user-friendly "build your own" instructions so you can buy just what you need.

My Computer Shopping List: Chips, RAM, and Burners

Parameters such as chip speed (how fast your data are exchanged), hard drive (HD) size (how much data you can store), RAM (random access memory, basically, how many instructions can be handled by the machine at once), and CD (compact disc) driver type are language basics you use to pick out your computer. If you are not computer literate or are just computer-challenged, don't be ashamed. Ask for help if you need it.

The computer is the backbone of your data collection and maintenance. You need reliability, quality, and user friendliness. Most systems come with a warranty. For example, most Dell systems have an in-house three-year service warranty. Grab that deal! However, don't get taken with a 10-year warranty when the world knows that computers stay current for only about three to four years, then need either upgrading or replacement.

The following minimum hardware parameters would serve you well:

- **2.0 MHz or greater speed chip**
- **80 gig HD**
- **512 MB RAM**
- **CD R/W (read/write) drive**

Innovations take place daily, so keep up with what's available by reading *Consumer Reports*™ and other computer and office supply magazines that will give you straightforward information on what you really need for your applications.

Save Me! (and My Data Too, Please)

You need the ability to save your data on a regular basis and, in the beginning, you can back up your data to a CD with your CD burner. When your business grows like wildflowers, you can

54   Starting & Managing Your Own Physical Therapy Practice

always add an external HD device to back up more extensive data. Newer "data sticks" (Sony calls them Memory Sticks™) can store 8MB to 128MB of information. By comparison, a CD holds about 700MB of data. Data sticks, each smaller than a stick of chewing gum, are sufficient for saving Word files and a limited number of documents or graphics. Data are transferred easily with a click of the mouse. The sticks are portable and slip easily into a pocket. Assuming you will develop a decent sized caseload relatively quickly, the "stick" will not be sufficient for your billing and patient demographic storage needs.

Your accountant should also be familiar with your require-ments because he or she uses computers to compile your taxes and generate your reports.

From the software perspective, your professional journals ad-vertise billing and business software geared specifically for phys-ical therapists. Billing systems exist for all sizes of practices, from the smallest one-man-show to well staffed, multi-site organiza-tions. The key is to select the most appropriate system. They all have 800 numbers and free demo disks to demonstrate what their capabilities are. Some offer not only patient data manage-ment and billing, but also have scheduling modules and patient tracking possibilities. There are two or three big players in our software market but, interestingly, I have always been more suc-cessful using a medical office package built for physicians and having the company tailor it for physical therapy (different cod-ing, etc). Be prepared to sink some substantial dollars into the software and yearly maintenance support fee. A ballpark figure for software purchase is $2,500 to $3,000 with an annual $500 to $1,000 support fee, which allows you unlimited toll-free calls to their support line when you (not IF you) run into snags.

Before you buy, ask the company for references, that is, oth-ers who use their software. Call every one of them to be sure you are dropping your cash into the right pocket. Fly by night, unknown companies who offer free hardware with their soft-ware and 20 years of free support are not recommended.

Get Booking! Computerized or Manual Scheduling?

There are pros and cons for both formats. Especially starting out, a manual schedule book will minimize computer confusion and keep everything in front of your eyes. I prefer a schedule book that shows the whole week in a glance, as opposed to flipping pages to see individual days. Most of our patients schedule appointments three times a week, and with a weekly book format, you have a direct view of what time slot may be open for all three visits. This makes it less confusing for the patients and minimizes the potential for the dreaded no-show!

On the other hand, getting used to a computerized scheduling system from the get-go is a benefit for organization too. When you are computerized, if a patient cancels with the flu, you can easily pull up his or her name and cancel all upcoming appointments without, for example, missing his or her Thursday appointment and losing out on the time slot that someone else could have filled. Computerization of the schedule also easily allows you to track your daily visits, cancellations, and no-shows without manually counting through scratch-outs, smears, and coffee stains on the schedule book.

Computerized scheduling usually comes as a module with any billing software package you buy. Support and training are included with the package. Alternately, you can buy a stand-alone computerized scheduler that does anything and everything as it relates to patient scheduling, including a tie in to the telephone to call the patient the night before to remind him or her of an appointment! I highly recommend PDS Solutions, an easy-to-use, powerful, and affordable software program for clinical documentation and scheduling (*www.PDSSolutions.com*).

 Be prepared: Transitioning to a computerized scheduling program from a manual system is usually fraught with resistance just because it is a newfangled format. It also seems much easier than it really is. If you need it, get help. Most software packages come with toll-free telephone support. Make sure you use it. Personally, I'd choose a computerized scheduling package to begin with just for the benefit of the patient tracking mechanism.

Electronic Reporting: The Future is Now!

The status quo for most private practice physical therapists are handwritten initial examination reports, dictated letters to referring practitioners with results of the examination and intervention plans, and hastily scribbled daily SOAP or narrative chart note documentation. The dictated reports either have to be transcribed in-house or sent out to a transcription service. Not only is this a costly way to get reports typed; it is also very time-consuming. You would be hard-pressed to get a dictated report in your hands to be proofread, sent back for corrections, re-typed, re-read for accuracy, put in an envelope, and sent out in the mail to the referral source in less than several days, right? Sometimes a week went by before letters that I had dictated came back for the initial proofreading. Also, writing notes by hand is time-consuming, has inherent error potential, is rarely standardized between clinicians, and is costly. (Remember: time is money!)

As technology improves, the concept of an electronic medical record (EMR) will become a reality for all healthcare providers, including physical therapists. Insurers and case managers for all the right reasons demand concise, clear, and informative reports documenting why their insured patient requires the services you are providing. With the insurance carriers investigating and scrutinizing written notes and reports to verify the medical necessity for your treatment, now, more than ever, your notes must objectively show that medical need.

Electronic reporting is quite beneficial for the provider for many reasons. Undecipherable handwriting will become clear, readable text. There will no longer be a need to stand at the copy machine reproducing daily notes to submit with the bill for reimbursement. Perhaps most importantly, time and money will be saved using a mechanized system of note dictation and report documentation, freeing time for you to treat patients.

The advent of personal computers, laptops, and PDAs has simplified the way in which you can collect and report your findings. There are numerous software companies on the market that sell and support both voice recognition and computerized programs that allow you to either speak your reports, design a template for commonly used reports, or use pull down menus to click and paste words, phrases, or frequently used paragraphs into a ready-to-send report.

If there was only a way to standardize reports and notes, have them miraculously appear on the computer screen in real time as we speak the words, and print them out in seconds. Well there is a way!

Voice recognition software (VRS) is a powerful tool that transforms the spoken word into written text in real time. Scansoft (*www.scansoft.com*) markets the most popular VRS, called Dragon NaturallySpeaking®. Using natural, everyday speech and talking to your computer to automate common tasks, customize and integrate applications, and turn your speech directly into text helps you work smarter and faster than ever before! You can dictate into virtually any Windows®-based application; navigate the Internet; perform speech-based text searches; and create and complete speech-aware document templates and forms with voice macros. Dragon Naturally-Speaking® Professional Solutions uses the power of speech to create, format, and edit documents, as well as to launch and control most desktop applications. Believe it or not, once loaded on your computer, Dragon has a very short learning curve. After 15 minutes of training (you simply read prepared text into a microphone and the software learns your voice and word pronunciation), the computer will get most of your spoken words correct, assuming you have the right equipment. When (not if) you plan on moving toward automated documentation of one sort or another, you must upgrade your computer's hardware system. VRS requires the minimum of a 500MHz Pentium III processor, 256 MB of RAM, and 300 MB of free hard drive space. However, the word on the street is that a Pentium 4 with 512 MB of RAM is preferable and more accurate in transforming the spoken word to the written text. In addition, a quality microphone (I use the Philips SpeedMike Pro microphone from *www.dictation.philips.com/na*) is highly recommended. Dragon VRS comes with a large medical vocabulary dictionary and can be used to dictate narrative letters to referring physicians or completing a pre-created note template.

Multiple therapists can share the software on one computer by simply clicking on the "voice profile" button on the screen. Of course, each user must train the software to recognize his or her own voice.

Lunis Orcutt, creator of KnowBrainer software (*www.knowbrainer.com*), has taken Dragon VRS a step further. Initially developed to assist the physically challenged and those with repetitive motion injuries, KnowBrainer is an easy-to-use, very extensive and sophisticated system of voice command macros, available for use in conjunction with Dragon System's voice command/dictation programs. Simplifying and condensing over 10,000 commands, applying basic common sense to produce optimal results with minimal effort, the KnowBrainer add-on makes using your computer hands-free.

So what's it all cost? Well, Lunis sells KnowBrainer and Dragon for less than what Scansoft sells Dragon itself for. With an investment of less than $750, you can get KnowBrainer and Dragon and be up and running in a weekend of set-up and training. If you are a computernik, it may even be shorter. Another advantage of dealing with Lunis is that the tech support is from Lunis himself. He answers the phone when you call and addresses your requests personally. He was very helpful each time I called and that service is a rarity nowadays.

Another excellent option in computerized record and note keeping is the use of templates with manual data entry and the use of pre-loaded field drop down menus to complete a form, report, or letter. With this format, the clinician sits at the keyboard and, using keystrokes and mouse clicks, he or she enters the patient's name and other demographics, history, physical findings, and interventions in standardized fields. There are many such programs currently on the market. I have found that PDS Solutions (*www.pdssolutions.com*) is the easiest and most intuitive program out there. PDS Solutions was developed by physical therapists in collaboration with an IT engineer. The software is proprietary to our profession and is very user-friendly. Navigation from fill-in-the-blank fields and drop-down menus is simple and sensible. Compared to VRS, manual data entry in the provided macro templates may be more time-consuming; however, I find a big advantage in having the fields pre-set before me when I sit down to compose a report or a daily clinic progress note. The template fields cue the clinician in a specified format lending to ease of use, standardization, speed, and accuracy. The therapist will not be prone to omit any area of the examination when the fields are right before his or her eyes. Besides the ease of use, PDS Solutions software is your best bet to complete, cost-effective, time saving, and accurate reporting.

In summary, choose VRS or manual data entry templates to computerize your reports and record keeping, and save yourself time and money!

Charge It! The **Plastic Fantastique**

While discussing automation, I must include the importance of obtaining and advertising your acceptance of credit cards for patient co-pay and bill payment at the front desk. Nearly all patients have some financial responsibility for their care and some welcome the convenience of paying their bills with credit cards. Some patients have up to a 30% co-insurance per visit. That can amount to $30 to $50 a visit! To accept payment by credit card, you must contact one of many companies that offer this service to merchants (that's you). Banks and other financial institutions supply you with a card swiper and charge a fee for each transaction performed. Most professional offices accept the two major cards, MasterCard™ and Visa™. Others may also accept American Express™ and Discover™. The more cards you choose to accept, the higher the fees are. Since most individuals primarily use Visa and MasterCard, one can safely say that accepting these payers is more than sufficient.

From an equipment standpoint, you'll need a regular electric outlet to plug in the swiper and receipt printer as well as a telephone jack to plug in the line for the swiper to transmit your payment information to the bank or intermediary. Most banks and many finance companies sell or lease credit card swipers with all kinds of bank terms. Your local Yellow Pages list them under "Credit Card Merchants." Some have a heavier up-front load to lease the machine and offer minimal percentages deducted for each transaction. Other companies lease the hardware for pennies and charge a larger percentage from each transaction. Weigh your options and know your numbers. You can also take the frugal route, most times more complicated but money saving in the long run, and click on *www.cheapcardswipers.com* or *www.swipers.com* for refurbished equipment and management deals.

 In this day and age, you need the availability of accepting credit cards or you stand to lose the "over the counter" payment and resort to billing the patient, extending the time the payment is not in your account. Always remember what experienced businessmen know as gospel: The longer you wait to collect money owed to you, the smaller the chance you will actually collect the money. Collecting co-pay, co-insurance, or deductible money owed to you with a credit card payment is almost as good as cash. Your only write-off is the one or two percentage point fee you pay the credit card company for the convenience of using its services.

Equipment Galore: How Do I Know What to Explore?

You've decided on your location, space needs, and niche market, now what on earth do you need to stock your new place? As with almost every question you have considered already, it depends. It depends on what type of practice you are creating. Will it be a general practice or a specialty practice?

Shoulda, Coulda, Woulda: The Equipment Tango

Let's divide the discussion into equipment you must have, should have, and wish you could have.

◆ **Must Have:** Every practice needs a front desk for the receptionist, chart file cabinets, a phone system, a telephone answering machine, a desk for the therapist, treatment tables, and modalities. In a general practice, begin with an ultrasound machine, an electrical stimulator of one sort or another, a hot pack machine, linens, pulleys, an overdoor traction device, a freezer, and a few weights. Assessment tools, such as a grip dynamometer, tape measure, reflex hammer, and a goniometer, are also a must.

- ◆ **Should Have:** A practice should have exercise equipment including a bike, a treadmill, free weights, cuff weights, Theraband, and some inflatable therapy balls. A washer/dryer makes life easier, more convenient, and cheaper in the long run. Running out of clean towels on a busy day is a nightmare. Remember you need to vent your dryer and have a 220V dedicated outlet for it.

- ◆ **Wish You Could Have:** The optimum scenario would be to have the following: whirlpool, mat tables, isokinetic assessment and training equipment (Cybex™, Kin-Com™, Biodex™, etc), cable column, upper body ergometer, iontophoresis stimulator, biofeedback, traction table, paraffin bath, and weight stack equipment.

Face the Music

Who would think that music is so important in the formula? Well, when you are evaluating Mrs. Smith and she is spilling her guts about her recent hysterectomy and slob of a husband, your other patient, Mr. Baloney, relaxing behind curtain number two on moist heat and electrical stimulation, should not be hearing this conversation. It turns out that music, set at a moderate level, keeps things in check. The music, set just loud enough to drown out Mrs. Smith's gynecologic history details, helps keep things confidential up to a point. In addition, almost all telephone system units (called key system units) have an input jack to run your stereo system through the phone main brain so that patients kept on hold can hum along with their favorite radio tunes. People placed on hold by your busy secretary should feel that you are still on the other end planning on getting to them soon. The "music on hold" system tends to make people feel that "you'll be with them soon," and it lends a bit to the professionalism of the office as well. Buy an AM/FM tuner from a local electronics retailer like Best Buy or Radio Shack®, a few ceiling tile-mounted speakers, some speaker wire, and you are set. The tuner will set you back less than $200, the speakers run about $50 each, and speaker wire goes for $10 per 50 foot spool. Installation is a snap in a drop ceiling (most office suites have dropped ceilings so you can run all kinds of wiring out of the public's view). Of course, for the maximum hush-hush, strategically placed solid walls are the most helpful in maintaining privacy and confidentiality.

Hello, Hello, Hello: Anyone Home?

Even before thinking about scheduling patients, you'll need to think about how the potential new customer will reach you. Consider keeping all options available: telephone, fax, e-mail, and snail mail. Your promotional materials should certainly list all the contact numbers you have to make the customer contact easier and problem-free.

Ring, Ring Ring...How Can One Person Answer Two Lines At Once? (and Other Problems You Hope to Have)

You have basically two options when it comes to phones: Buy standard one, two, or three line phones from retailers like Best Buy or Circuit City® or buy a system from your local phone line service provider (for example, Verizon® in Maryland) or a private telephone contractor. Check your local Yellow Pages for telephone company listings. You'll find plenty of choices.

 If you are handy, you may want to save a bundle and wire the new office yourself. You'll be surprised how easy it is to run telephone cable through drop ceilings and cut holes in the drywall to mount the telephone jack box. There are two types of modern telephone cable: "four pair" or "category five." Four pair is a cable that has eight total wires color-coded to hook up four telephone lines. As you have surmised, each phone line takes two wires to connect. Category five cable also has four pairs of wires to allow four phone lines to be installed, but the sets of wires are twisted in a special fashion to minimize hum and interference. Category five, also nicknamed "Cat-5," is primarily used for networking computers, but I use it for all my communications needs.

If you hire a contractor to run your wiring, it'll cost you about $50 to $75 an hour. To wire a 1,500 square foot suite with three phone lines and, say, five phone jacks, will run you about $500.

Unless you are truly a techno-geek, you'll need a technician to install a base unit for your telephone system. No doubt you'll want all the features of a good phone system, including music on hold, intercom capabilities, and message taking when you are unavailable. Telephone systems with a base station and five multi-line phones will run about $2,500. Check out the following websites for system information: *http://www.toshiba.com/taistsd/pages/prd_dk_main.html*, *http://www.panasonic.com/consumer_electronics/telephones/default.asp*, *www.thephoneconnection.com*, and *www.telephonesystems.com*.

For those of you who are brave, pioneering souls and have good hands, you may buy the whole telephone system, wiring, calibration and all, online and install it yourself. The systems come with illustrated installation manuals and run anywhere from $750 into the thousands. As an example, check out this site: *www.leephones.com*.

Used systems are readily available as well. I would recommend a good service contract if you want to go used. Two used phone system sites are *www.usedphones.com* and *http://www.etelephonesystems.com/systems.htm*. You'll also find used telephone dealers and installers in your local Yellow Pages.

Uh Oh! No One's Home

You'll have to be sure that you have a system in place to answer your calls when you are not in the office or when you and your small staff are busy. The cheapest and easiest way to handle the incoming calls you can't grab that second (you should be so lucky!) is to purchase an inexpensive (less than $75) telephone answering machine and tape a kind message in a sweet voice stating how much you would have loved to answer their call, but you are busy helping another patient at this time. The message should of course state the name of the business, the phone number, the days the business is open, and the hours of operation. The machine can be checked for messages upon your staff's arrival every morning or even from a remote location. Another option for an answering system is to use the phone company's internal answering service. This system automatically transfers your caller to the voice mail when you are not in the office, unavailable, or on another line. When messages are left on voice mail, you are alerted by a series of beeps when you lift the receiver to make a call. You can check in anytime in the office or from a remote location as well. My vote would be to go with voice mail. That way, you never lose a call even when you are on the line(s).

Vision is the art of seeing the invisible.

—*Jonathan Swift*

CHAPTER 8

Caring about Medicare

Should I Care about Medicare?

What is Medicare and do I need to be in some way connected to this mammoth? Medicare is a federally funded and managed health insurance plan for senior citizens over age 65, some people younger than 65 with disabilities, and people with end-stage renal disease. The Medicare program is divided into two parts: Part A and Part B. Part A covers inpatient care in hospitals, skilled nursing facilities, and fees for some home care agencies. Part B helps cover part of physicians' services and outpatient hospital bills. It also covers medically necessary physical and occupational therapy services, which is why *you should care about Medicare*! For specific information, see the handbook entitled "Medicare and You" at *www.medicare.gov*. This handbook offers extensive information about the Medicare system and benefits.

 As an aside, many, if not most, other health care organizations ask if you are a credentialed Medicare provider prior to even beginning to negotiate with you to be a preferred provider with them. Most carriers will not even entertain your interest in them if you are not a credentialed Medicare provider. And so it goes...

Medicare: What's in It for Me?

The decision as to whether you should become a provider with Medicare or not is related to the caseload you choose to treat in your practice. Most practices have a nice chunk of Medicare beneficiaries in their coffers since most of the elderly population has a distinct need for the services physical therapists provide. As a credentialed provider, Medicare pays you directly, avoiding the hassle and headache of billing your patients after they have received the Medicare check weeks or months later. Once you agree to be a Medicare provider, you consent to accept payment that Medicare deems "usual and customary."

That Custom Is Unusual

Usual and Customary (U+C) means that Medicare chops your bill down to what it believes is acceptable for the time you spent treating the patient and in what geographic location you provided the services. As a Medicare provider, you agree to accept the U+C amount as your full fee for services rendered and pledge not to *balance bill* your patient for the noncovered amount. Balance bill means that you have agreed to accept Medicare's U+C amount as your billed amount and, in return, Medicare pays you quickly and directly (when you electronically bill them), providing you and the patient with an easy to read explanation of benefits.

Can You Cap This?

The government has attempted to harness Medicare spending over the past decade or so. One method Congress decided upon was to limit outpatient physical therapist in independent practice (PTIP) reimbursement for Medicare beneficiaries. In the mid-1990s, the maximum amount Medicare would pay for its patients treated in a PTIP was $1,500 annually. This $1,500 severely cut into patients' benefits and forced the therapists involved to keep a close tally on their Medicare patients' bills. Due to the reimbursement restrictions imposed by Congress, patients were often discharged before their maximum benefit from therapy was achieved. The cap was rescinded a few years later after much protest by therapists and patient advocates. They asked that Congress study the numbers better and calculate what the government paid for benefits for patients seen in a PTIP compared to therapy provided in a hospital-based outpatient setting, a physician-owned physical therapy clinic, and corporate-owned practices. I am not convinced that any formal study of benefit reimbursements was made by Congress in the years after the first moratorium, but in another desperate attempt at control the upward spiral of Medicare payments paid to providers, Congress in 2002 placed a $1,590 cap on outpatient physical therapy, this time including all providers except hospital-based (Medicare Part A) centers. With extensive lobbying efforts, Congress in 2003 again placed a moratorium on the $1,590 cap, thereby allowing Medicare recipients unlimited therapy benefits based upon documented medical necessity. Keeping up with Medicare regulations is a relatively simple but very critical task for the private practice owner. The American Physical Therapy Association (APTA) website (*www.apta.org*) keeps a vigilant eye on reimbursement issues, as does the APTA's Private Practice Section (*www.ppsapta.org*). It is incumbent upon all physical therapists to be informed of reimbursement issues that affect us in all we do.

What's an EOB?

An EOB is a list of services you provided, notation of what Medicare (or any other payer) deems OK to charge, their adjustment trimmed off of your submitted fee, how much they are paying you, and how much you can legally bill the patient.

OK, OK—I Surrender: I'll Become a Medicare Provider

How do you take the leap of faith and become a flag-waving Medicare provider? To become a Medicare provider, you must request an application packet, a virtual encyclopedia of all kinds of questions, names, addresses, and other pertinent data, directly from your Medicare carrier (also called an intermediary). Every state or region contracts with Medicare via a local carrier, that is, a company that goes between the provider and customer (patient) and Medicare, the federal government agency. For example, in Maryland, the local carrier is Trailblazer (*http://www.trailblazerhealth.com*). Your local carrier will review your application and, assuming everything is in order, will issue you a provider number. In most cases the process takes about six weeks. Any errors or incomplete information on the application will cause delays. The carrier processes your application, future claims, and other clerical issues. So then who pays the bills? A fiscal intermediary pays your submitted bills. In Maryland, the fiscal intermediary is Carefirst of Maryland or Mutual of Omaha (depending in which part of Maryland your office is located). You may quickly and easily locate your region, carrier, and fiscal intermediary by setting your Internet browser to *http://cms.hhsgov/providers/enrollment/contacts/* and enter your state.

Why this hubbub about applying for Medicare? Because you most likely need a Medicare provider number to work with other carriers, commercial and otherwise, and it takes at least six weeks to land the golden number of opportunity. So, until you receive a provider number from your local Medicare carrier, your services will not be considered "qualified" and/or "covered" services by Medicare.

In other words, while your training and experience might otherwise meet the qualifications to become a Medicare provider, unless you have actually applied for and received a Medicare provider number, your services will not be paid by Medicare. Because local Medicare carriers and their numbers tend to change frequently, the Centers for Medicare and Medicaid Services website is your best source for accurate, up-to-date information. Keep updated by logging onto *http://cms.hhs.gov/contacts/incardir.asp*.

Call the carrier in your state to verify its procedure for obtaining a Medicare provider number. By the way, Medicare pays 80% of the U+C amount. That means that if you bill Medicare $100 for your services on Mr. Johnson and Medicare says that the U+C fee is $80, Medicare will chip in $64 (80% of $80) and you must chase Mr. Johnson for the $16 balance due. Many people have Medi-Gap policies or secondary payers that pick up what Medicare doesn't pay, but don't be fooled. Mr. Johnson's secondary policy only pays the 20% figure of $16 and you have to adjust off the $20 that Medicare terms unusual and noncustomary! Happy chasing.

Another Headache: Medicaid. Must I Care about That, Too?

Medicaid is a jointly funded, federal-state health insurance program for certain low-income and needy people. It covers approximately 36 million Americans including children, the aged, blind, and/or disabled, and people who are eligible to receive federally assisted income maintenance payments. Medicaid is also called Medical Assistance. They maintain a fee schedule, which means they have a list of what they will pay you by the modality or procedure you bill. Generally, their payments are well below U+C amounts and some, if not many, therapists choose not to be a provider. Further information on Medicaid is located at *http://cms.hhs.gov/medicaid/*

We don't accomplish anything in this world alone...and whatever happens is the result of the whole tapestry of one's life and all the weavings of individual threads from one to another that creates something.

—*Sandra Day O'Connor*

CHAPTER 9

Marketing Magic

Shouldn't I Think about Where My Patients Will Come From?

Now that the planning is done, where will patients come from? I naively thought that once I hung my shingle outside the office door and sent a bundle of brochures announcing the opening of my new practice to a few area doctors, patients would be clamoring to come in and see me. Why wouldn't they? Didn't I believe that I was qualified, had a spanking new facility, was eager to please each and every patient that visited me, and had the ability to heal all their pains?

Sadly, nothing could have been further from the truth. As a business owner, you must make marketing a priority in doing business, an effort to build and promote long-term relationships with your customers. What is marketing and how does it pertain to everything you do in a day's work? Read on to find out….

Off to **Market**

Customer service. In my mind, that is the definition of marketing. Marketing attracts customers, draws them into a business, and keeps them there. Let's recall who the customers are. Your four customers include the referring practitioner, the patient himself, the patient's insurance carrier, and your staff. Customers today demand choice, flexibility, quality, high levels of service, and expect that businesses respond to their preferences rapidly. To be and stay successful, you must respond to a customer's multiple needs and requirements. You need a plan!

What about Creating a Marketing Plan Now?

You need a plan to draw in and satisfy your customer. A marketing plan helps you establish, direct, and coordinate your marketing efforts. It is often a component of your business plan. Preparing a marketing plan forces you to assess what's going on in your marketplace and how it affects your business. It also provides a benchmark for later measurement. Often, simply embarking on the process of preparing a marketing plan guides you in developing a successful marketing strategy. The marketing plan helps you identify exactly who your customer is, promote the culture of your business, and build lasting relationships with your customers (in this case, with your referring practitioners and payers). When you prepare to write your marketing plan, think like the customer. What do you offer that the practice down the road doesn't? What gaps can you fill in that your competitors have missed? Your plan should include everything you do to create awareness of your practice and your goals and strategies of building that awareness. Who are your targeted customers? When I opened my practice in an area of scarce potential referral sources, I re-identified my customers as those who live and work in a heavily populated area that for some reason didn't have many medical providers. Therefore, I had to market to my potential referring practitioners and convince them that I was their "preferred Western County provider of quality, personalized physical therapy care." I was not the practitioner's neighborhood therapist but rather their man in the western area of the county where their patients worked or lived.

How Do I Drag the Patients through the Door?

How will anyone know you actually exist? Hanging a shingle on the front lawn used to work, but no more. You have to promote yourself! You must create an awareness of your services to your target population. Marketing your name and your practice is much more than "selling." Michael Porter, one of the foremost leaders in marketing research, writes that marketing is the process of planning, designing, and developing products and services, including pricing, promotion, and the distribution of products and services, to the customer. The owner must identify the customer's need and then fill that need. How, you ask? Well, the three methods of promotion according to the marketing gurus are *personal selling*, *public relations*, and *advertising*. Examples of each are as follows:

- ◆ **Personal selling** is what many of us are pretty good at doing— Hitting a doctor up for patient referrals with a firm handshake and a wink. Our success is based on our ability to go out and hustle up business, beating our own drum, and making others feel welcome. I try to create an image of value for my customers. I want them to know what I represent in my professional and ethical pursuit of excellence, my high quality of service at a fair price, my attention to customer service, and my dedication to the patient's overall well-being.
- ◆ **Public relations** is the business of inventing and molding a corporate image of your practice and your staff. It is also the method of selling yourself using various media such as TV, radio, the Internet, and billboards.
- ◆ **Advertising** is using hard goods to inform potential customers of your business. It can take the form of brochures, logos, business cards, or prescription pads.

When you see a potential referral source at a local high school sports event and hand him a business card, is that personal selling or public relations? Is it advertising or personal selling? What's the difference? If it brings patients through the door, celebrate your marketing success!

What advertising media will you employ to get the word out? Design and maintain your own website? Yellow Pages' advertising? Billboard displays? Brochure mailings? Bagel breakfasts to potential local referral sources? These are all great ideas, but you have to consider the pros and cons of each. Your marketing plan will better focus your ideas and their practicality.

Develop your marketing plan by writing short-term (six months) and long-term (one to two years) objectives since the plan takes time to play out in the long run. Identify segments of your general population by geographic location, residence, or employment; managed care or commercial insurance coverage; work type; diagnosis type; ethnic background; gender; or avocation interests. To start with, compose a simple, one paragraph marketing plan that includes:

- ◆ **What** will the plan accomplish?
- ◆ **How** will the plan help and/or satisfy the customer?
- ◆ **Who** is the customer?
- ◆ **What** is the business?
- ◆ **What** need does the business fulfill (what is the company's niche)?
- ◆ **How** will the word get out? What media will you use to advertise?
- ◆ **What** will it cost to get the word out?

Promote Thyself!

Promotion is the creative side of marketing that includes advertising, publicity, and personal selling. The mode you choose to use to get your name out to the proper channels is called the "promotional mix." Get input from others as to the most economic and effective way to get your name in front of those who can help keep you busy. Many physical therapists spend huge sums on promoting their practices.

My Own Tricks

I have found that getting my letterhead on the desk of referring practitioners has been my most useful promotional tool. Take any opportunity to send a letter to a referring practitioner (it costs less than a dollar a letter and is very effective).

- ◆ **When a patient is referred by a specialist (an orthopedist, rheumatologist, or physiatrist), I ask the patient for his or her primary care physician's name. That doctor gets a copy of the report too.**
- ◆ **Am I adding staff? I send out a letter. Am I extending hours to accommodate the working patient population? I send out a letter. Here's an example:**

Dear Dr. Johnson:

This is to inform you that we have extended our patient care hours till 7 P.M. Monday through Friday for the convenience of the working patient.

As always, you can count on us to provide quality and personalized care to your patients any time of the day.

Feel free to call should you have further questions.

◆ **Did the practitioner just make the business section of the newspaper because she became director of the department? I send out a letter.**

The more letters, the better. That is what is called "name recognition" or "brand recognition" in the business lexicon. Until they fell asleep at the wheel and ran into major competition in the late 1990s, don't you think Levi's was smart to sew that little red tag on the back pocket of their jeans since the 1890s? Who didn't think of Levi's when they thought of blue jeans? Why does Hershey place their name in large, bold letters across their product, but write the words "chocolate bar" in a much smaller font size? That is so every time you need a chocolate fix, you'll think of Hershey and not Nestle or another brand. Hershey taught us to think of a "Hershey bar" instead of a "chocolate bar." What about Kleenex® and Jell-O®? These are brand names you'll never forget.

So, your promotional goal is for the referring practitioner to think YOUR NAME whenever the words "physical therapy" cross his or her mind. Then, your marketing goal is to have him or her smile, reach for a pen and prescription pad, and write the referral to you.

How Do I Get My Hands on the Gold? Who Has the List?

You would never believe it but another entrepreneur had the same questions and came up with an idea. An internist, Dr. Jerry Spitz, decided to collate a list of area physician names, specialties, addresses, and contact numbers in a handy little book that other physicians and people like us could use for marketing purposes. In 1988, Dr. Spitz founded the Little Blue Book Company that publishes these little guides, distributing them in 146 metropolitan areas with pharmaceutical company sponsorship. For those who are more tech-savvy, the book even comes in a PDA and PC version. The company's mission is to help practicing physicians provide better patient care by providing practical tools that simplify their daily tasks. Since doctors themselves actually use their Little Blue Book, they make sure all of their information is up-to-date, making the database of practicing physicians more accurate and complete than any other database. I can't tell you how wonderful this little book is. For $15 a copy, you can't lose. Order one by simply logging onto *http://www.thelittlebluebook.com*. Another method of gaining access to physician lists in your metro area is by contacting the local chapter of your city's medical society. They are usually happy to sell you a listing or even mailing labels of member physicians for a hefty cost.

The world is divided into people who do things and people who get the credit; opt to belong to the first class, there's far less competition.

—*Dwight Morrow*

CHAPTER 10

Advertising and Promotion

Stationery, Forms, and Promotional Materials: Who Sells What?

Your basic printed materials will include a letterhead, envelopes with your name and return address embossed in the corner, business and appointment cards, prescription pads, and promotional materials such as brochures or novelty materials (printed key fobs, Rolodex® cards, embossed mugs, and the like). Check out the Appendix for sample forms.

Here is a rundown of what you need:

◆ **Letterhead:** Logo or not, you should have a simple yet classy letterhead motif listing the company name, address, phone and fax numbers, e-mail address, website (if you have one), and staff.

◆ **Business cards:** Cards should be printed for each and every staff member who has direct contact with the customer, including professional staff and the business manager or office coordinator. Give out your business cards freely. They act as great marketing awareness tools to practitioners and customers alike. Local printers are listed in your Yellow Pages or on the Internet.

◆ **Promotional materials:** Materials may include novelty items like coffee mugs and paper pad cubes embossed with your name, logo, or anything that will put your company's identity in the referral source's mind. Printing Rolodex cards is a great way to keep your name at the practitioner's or his or her staff's fingertips. Everyone has a Rolodex file system on their desk, right? Printing 250 Rolodex cards costs about $200 plus setup charges. Print them in a bold and bright color so they'll stand out every time the individual flips through the cards.

◆ **Prescription pads:** These pads are a very valuable marketing tool to keep your name, address, and phone number under the referral source's nose. Use the same header design that you employ on your letterhead to keep things standard in the minds of your referral sources. List the treatment modalities and procedures you offer, leaving space for the referring practitioner to sign the form and add other pertinent information he or she wants you to know about the patient. The printer can create them in any number of sheets you want. Use bright, bold colors to keep your pad more visible than your competitor's. My pads are printed on bright yellow stock with black ink. I typically order 50 pads of 20 sheets each.

♦ **Appointment cards:** Besides letterhead, envelopes, business cards, and prescription pads, don't forget to order appointment cards to use when you schedule your patients. Unlike everything said about sharp designs and attractive logos, for appointment cards, get the simplest and cheapest black and white card available. They are throwaways that patients usually lose anyway and have no marketing afterlife.

Where Do I Get All This Printed and Monogrammed Stuff?

Printed Material

I do all my printing (forms, letterhead, envelopes, business cards, appointment cards, brochures, and prescription pads) at local print shops like Sir Speedy or Kinko's and get 24-hour turnaround, free pickup and delivery, and bulk discounts for larger orders. For brochures, they will set up the entire publication and charge you for their time or you can bring camera-ready layout and they will print it for you. *Camera ready* (also called *wysiwyg*, which stands for "**w**hat **y**ou **s**ee **i**s **w**hat **y**ou **g**et") means that the print shop will print exactly what you hand them. Check for typos, smudges, smears, etc. Software like Microsoft Publisher© and other graphics packages have brochure layout wizards. They are very user-friendly and will give you creative license to make an attractive, promotional publication that is camera ready. Pricing and other assorted fees can be found on the print shop's website such as *www.kinkos.com* or *www.sirspeedy.com*. In fact, you can even send your printing layout to them online and they can produce the materials and deliver them to you. I am not sure that these two companies are the cheapest way to go, but I have found them to be very reliable and competitive. They will match competitors' prices.

Promotional Advertising

For promotional advertising, I order embossed novelty materials right off the Internet. Set your browser to "advertising ideas and promotional novelties," and you'll see tons of sites. I have used *www.imprintproducts.com* and found them easy to work with and free with creative ideas. Another site is *www.advertising-novelties.com*, which lists a multitude of contacts for personalized promotional novelty gifts.

An interesting Internet site, Vista Print, offers limited volume, free business card printing, using one of their clever, colorful, eye-catching templates. Check them out at *www.vistaprint.com*. They are free (sans shipping at a cost of about $6 for 250 cards) because Vista Print advertises its company's name in a nonobtrusive fashion on the back of your free card. You can order the cards without Vista Print's name for an extra fee, and also buy cards in a larger bulk at around $35 for 2,000 cards. I used them and I cannot tell you how many compliments I have received on these cards. Because they are multicolored and quite unusual, they tend to grab one's attention much more than the standard black and white mundane card. If you are different, show it in your design, layout, and creativity.

Make a Name for Yourself

Most importantly, your promotional materials must stand out, be different, and attract attention! One of your first decisions is whether you want or need a logo. It is costly to professionally create and produce a logo and is not totally necessary, yet many practices have one. The logo sets you apart and has the capacity in the customers' minds to identify you with a symbol. If you choose to have a logo, you may want to design it based on your name, corporate name, location, or expertise. Setting your Internet browser to "private physical therapy practices" will land you hundreds of hits. Click on a few to get ideas of what company logos look like and how you may create your logo with similar ideas. Many logos in our field are based on movement, recovery, sports, bright icons, colorful swooshes (similar to the Nike sneaker company's logo), and curlicues based on the company's name or initials. Here is my logo:

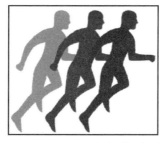

Figure 1. Sample company logo

ESTERSON
& ASSOCIATES
PHYSICAL THERAPY

I chose my logo to show movement (it's what we do!) and my font to be bold and dynamic. "Esterson" is in a larger font size for easier name recognition (remember our Hershey discussion) but "& Associates" and the words "physical therapy" are included as well.

Think about font styles and colors. A practice wanting to attract a female clientele may be better off with a thinner, curlier font in softer colors compared to a different font and color palate for a practice promoting sports medicine to college athletes. If you are not of the creative, artsy type, you can engage the services of a professional graphic designer. Depending on your budget, it may be cost effective to have the designer do all your stationery and other promotional material layouts and printing as well. As was mentioned earlier, try looking for a local university or art school that is interested in having one of its students create your logo and lay out your promotional products as a class project. Going that way will certainly be more cost effective. If you do decide on a logo, use it on all your advertising, letterhead, and business cards as a method of emblazoning your company ID upon your customers' minds.

Paperwork, Paperwork, Paperwork: What Forms Do I Need?

Besides your stationery, business cards, appointment cards, and prescription pads, you'll need various forms before you even open your doors for business. Take a peek at the Appendix. I've included all the forms for your perusal.

Think about the last time you saw your personal physician. You entered his office, signed in on an attendance form, gave your medical history while he wrote notes on an examination form, possibly took a prescription from him on a prescription sheet, and checked out with a super bill indicating what the doctor did for you that day. Similarly, you'll need forms tailored to what you do with your patients on any given day. Follow the same trail. You'll need:

◆ **A sign-in attendance form:** This form shows today's date, has a space for the patient's signature, and a space for the patient's appointment time. With Health Insurance Portability and Accountability Act (HIPAA) regulations (see Chapter 12) and patient privacy protection in mind, some offices use a cover sheet over the last patient's signature so the next patient signing in cannot see the others who signed in before him. Other practices are using sheets of peel off labels for their sign in sheets. Once the patient signs in, the receptionist peels off that label and affixes it to a secure paper out of the view of others.

◆ **An intake form:** This is the form the receptionist first fills out when a new patient calls to schedule. It includes the patient's name, address, phone number at home and work, date of birth, social security number, employer, reason for referral to physical therapy, insurance policy numbers, and other pertinent insurance information. There is also a section on the form for the billing clerk to complete the insurance verification process, that is, calling the payer and asking what benefits are available, what the co-pay or co-insurance amounts are, if there is a deductible and if it has been met for the year prior to the patient arriving for care.

◆ **An examination form:** You may want to use ideas from a form that you used in your hospital job or one you used as a student years ago. Perhaps you may want to redesign a combination of several forms you are familiar with. Be sure to use your logo and/or letterhead on the top of the form.

◆ **An encounter form or *Superbill*:** This is a sheet that lists all the possible diagnoses (ICD-9) and treatment (CPT) codes you may use on any patient in a given day with small checkoff boxes next to each code. Once these forms are completed by you or your staff, the billing department uses these forms to create a charge for the day's visit and generates the bill to the appropriate payer.

◆ **A fax cover sheet:** This is similar to your letterhead format but includes the following: fax to name, fax to number, regarding, number of pages faxed including the cover sheet, and a disclaimer paragraph to state that the information you fax may be confidential and is directed only to the person to whom the fax is sent.

◆ **HIPAA compliance form:** This is a required written description of your HIPAA privacy and security policies and notes the name and contact person of your compliance officer.

As with the other printed materials, you can design these yourself and take them to a local print shop, or the shop can prepare the layout, submit them for your approval, and then print and deliver the materials to you. Obviously, if you do the design and layout, you will save significant *moolah*.

How Will People Know I Am Open for Business?

Do I really need a flashing red neon sign that says: ***THERAPY HERE***? The choice of which methods you will employ to promote your new venture is called the "promotional mix." The promotional mix dictates where your advertising dollars will be spent. Consider advertising in the newspaper or even placing a public service news release that you have opened your new facility and cater to whatever niche market you have chosen. A listing in the Yellow Pages is a must for most practices. Who doesn't look for business addresses or phone numbers in the

Yellow Pages? The larger box ads are exponentially more expensive than the simple line listing. I don't believe that a large box ad gives a practitioner more business, since most of our referrals come directly from physicians and not from patients searching for the largest box ad in the Yellow Pages. I would agree though that a bold name listing is more impressive to the patient seeking your phone number than a plain font name listing. Some practices are developing their own websites. Although involved and somewhat costly to create and run, many realize that the public is now more computer-savvy and seeks out online information as a first information investigation method more than ever before. Radio spots reach a market that perhaps other print media do not. It's the same deal with TV. The bottom line is that you have to choose your advertising attack and let the world know you are ready!

Now here's what I did: My promotional mix included a bold listing in the city's metropolitan Yellow Pages, an online Yellow Page listing, and I swamped every local township and county newspaper and city-wide newspaper with multiple press releases. One press release announced the opening of our new facility on Rolling Road. Two weeks later another release went out announcing that I was personally opening a new outpatient physical therapy practice. A few months later when I brought on a staff physical therapist to join me, I again sent two releases to the area print media. One announced that I was pleased to welcome a new member to my team. The second emphasized our clinic's reputation for providing high quality and personalized service to the community, our new expanded hours with the addition of a highly qualified staff, and again a blurb about the new employee's impressive credentials. Get it? The more information the public sees and hears, the more "brand" recognition you get. Don't be fooled into thinking that every newspaper will print everything you send. Print media tend to chop and cut large pieces of what they feel is verbose and run-on information. Try to address what you believe the public needs to know: your name, your credentials, your reputation, your experience, your specialty, your location, your contact information, and any other blockbuster information that will impress the paper's editors and subsequent readership.

When I returned to practice after a 2-year sabbatical, I sent press releases to radio and TV stations in my listening and viewing areas. To my knowledge, neither ever broadcasted the announcement but, then again, it could have aired between 3 A.M. and 4 A.M. Who knows? With that said, I would not advise pursuing radio and TV spots as a rookie practice owner.

 If you are active in a church or synagogue, get the word out through its newsletter or through an announcement from the pulpit congratulating you on opening your new clinic. If you are a member of a civic or social organization, spread the word through its mailings. One of my most successful "get the word out" techniques was writing brief exercise and health-related articles for the local church and synagogue community. The religious organizations happily accepted my two or three paragraph informational article with my name, credentials, location, and contact numbers placed at the end of the article. For them, it was a great "filler" in their monthly bulletins and offered their readers useful information. It gave me free advertising. I negotiated that for my free advice, I would have my name and other information set in boldface type at the end of each article so it would jump out at the readers. In fact, patients who were referred by their physicians would comment that they read my article in their organization's newsletter *religiously*! In this fashion, I successfully built "brand recognition." I got my name out to a local target population (including the physicians who were members of that specific church or synagogue), developed recognition as an "author" and, in the readers' minds, I became "the expert." Even better, the patients returned to their physicians after my care and raved that not only did they receive superior attention and service at Esterson's clinic, but that I was also the author of the weekly health and fitness column in the St. Luke's Bulletin.

Your marketing plan will discuss how and to whom you will advertise and promote your business. After you define who your customers are (see prior information in Chapter 1 on identifying all four of your customers), develop your marketing strategy to meet their demands.

Realistically, the high majority of your patients are sent to you by referring practitioners or other satisfied customers. By and large, these practitioners are local private physicians, dentists, podiatrists, nurse practitioners, case managers, managed care group referral coordinators, or other patients you previously treated who thought you were the best thing since sliced bread.

From my point of view, I spend most of my advertising buck on being sure that this group knows who I am, where I am, and what I can do to help their referred patients. How do I do it? Well, as I mentioned previously, I bombard their respective desks with my letterhead for any and every possible reason. I may also attack from the north with a bagel breakfast for their staff and from the east with a promotional novelty like a coffee mug with my company name on it.

 I make it my business to come up with a creative and unforgettable gift item at holiday times. For example, one year, I gave my referring physicians a personalized coffee mug shaped like a big lumbar vertebra, a novelty item from the Anatomical Chart Company (*http://anatomical.com/item_disp.asp?PN= CMM-1*). They never forgot that gift and my business soared from one simple idea. The Internet has plenty of sites that will kick your imagination into gear. Lands' End, the well-known online clothing retailer, is now offering a business outfitters link. Log onto *www.landsend.com* and click on the tab that says "business outfitters" to see all kinds of merchandise that can be personalized with your company name and logo. The site is simple to navigate and even allows you to create a logo online! *Marty@imprintproducts.com* will give you free advice on using giveaways to promote your practice. And who doesn't like chocolate? Websites like *www.chocolatique.com* and *www.hersheygifts. com*, among others, create chocolate bars and gifts imprinted with your name and logo. Again, if you're not creative, it'll cost you, but plenty of companies are around to do the job for you, including delivery.

Billboards and Billfolds: Do I Need to Advertise My Venture?

Advertising, promotion, and selling have already been covered. So has the idea of spending money to make money. But what about mass advertising with an outdoor sign? It's costly but effective. You need to know that many professional parks have strict rules about uniformity of exterior signage. Similarly, the same type of building complexes may not allow interior signage on the windows. The reason for all of these rules is to maintain a standard in the building or buildings so that each tenant does not put up grossly oversized signs and clutter the exterior. A better reason is that the landlord often has a deal going with a particular sign company and directs all the tenants to use that company. Exterior signage can run into hundreds or thousands of dollars and even more if the sign is backlit (a more expensive, fancier sign that has a lighted background making the lettering and/or logo stand out). However, outside signage gets you noticed on a daily basis more than a listing in the Yellow Pages. Another benefit of an exterior sign is to direct your customers to your doorstep. This is especially important if, like me, you have more than one therapy clinic in your building. Your exterior sign gets the scheduled customer in your door where he or she belongs. No one wants to lose customers!

Set Your Sights on a Website

In today's world of cybertechnology, any discussion about getting your name out needs to include information about websites, and I strongly recommend including a website in your promotional mix. Your site should be clean, crisp, and informative without overwhelming the Web surfer with blinking and animated cartoons or other distractions. Include your name, address, locale, directions, specialties, target population, services provided, clinic photos, staff portraits and profiles, insurance participation, and links to other sites offering further information about what you do. A link to a description of your privacy policy and billing information is appropriate. Most sites have hyperlinks to e-mail you and your staff, making communication between you and your customers easy and immediate. Sadly, many current practices maintain less than appealing websites and have a sloppy and elementary appearance.

To begin creating your site, look at what your peers have already done. My suggestion would be to set your browser to "private physical therapy practices" and choose a few sites that you like. From there you can either use a software program, like Microsoft Front Page, Macromedia's Dreamweaver, or similar software, to create your own website. If such a concept scares you or if you are as creative as a tube of ultrasound gel, then there are loads of website designers who would love to help you create a simple site for your practice. Costs for professionals to design your site run anywhere from $250 to $1,500 depending on how many pages you want, how much glitz you choose, and basically, how much time it takes the professional designer to get your ideas computer-coded. Here are a few other possibilities you may want to try before engaging a Web designer:

1. Call a few local high schools or two-year colleges and ask for their computer department. Many computer teachers have a crackerjack, talented kid who is a prodigal expert in hypertext markup language (HTML) and JavaScript, the secret codes of website design. A friend of mine engaged a high school senior who is a whiz at web design and created a bright and functional site for his online promotional products business. The two agreed on $8 an hour and the kid knocked the project out in 25 hours! His 20-page site, full of photos and graphics, cost him only $200. Could you beat that? The student also agreed to maintain and manage the site (called being the site's "webmaster") and tweak it for him whenever necessary for a similar meager monthly fee.

2. The online behemoth bookseller, Amazon.com (*www. amazon.com*), offers all kinds of "build your own website" guides. I found that books like *Building a Website for Dummies* by Crowder and Crowder, *HTML for Dummies* by Tittel and James, and *The Complete Idiot's Guide to Creating a Web Page* by McFedries were very helpful when I created my own site. Check them out!

3. How Web Pages Work (*http://computer.howstuffworks.com/web-page.htm*) is a website that teaches you how to create, upload, and promote your own information. The site covers such topics as basic HTML formatting tags, creating frames and tables, uploading and setting up images, and promoting your site. Even if you are not inclined to cre-

ate your own site, the information on this site will give you the proper understanding and web-design jargon to intelligently discuss your ideas and plans with an experienced website designer.

In a nutshell, in order to get your website up and running, you need three things:

1. A domain name (the name entered when someone searches for you online, for example, EstersonTherapy.com or Friendship-PT.com)
2. An HTML and JavaScript-coded program called your web page or website
3. A host or server who will put your created program (website) on the Web and out to the world

Following the steps above, you first must create your virtual (site) name. There are literally hundreds of sites you can use to register your name. Try this one: log onto *www.register.com* to register your selected domain name. Don't be too wordy or complex. It will confuse your intended audience who wants to read about you and your product. Use a name that people can easily recall. Sometimes your chosen domain name has been taken by another company. Suppose your company is called Brockington Services. You log onto *www.register.com* to register your domain, and much to your chagrin you learn that Brockington Services is also the name of a company in another state that sells corned beef to take-out delis nationwide. If you wish to stick with your corporate name, then you may try BrockServ.com or Brockingtontherapyservices.com. Remember, do not be too wordy. You may also try the same name with a .net or .biz suffix. However, the pros I know tell me that companies should stick with the .com suffix since .com is what most people using the net are accustomed to seeing. I felt that estersonandassociatesphysicaltherapy.com was obviously way too tedious for a potential Web-surfing customer to type in his or her browser, so instead, I chose EstersonTherapy.com. As with all promotional and marketing attempts, my rule says that anything that may throw off the potential customer from reaching you is never recommended. Hyphenating and underlining between words, for example, Esterson-Therapy.com or Esterson_Therapy.com, according to my sources "in the know," is difficult for the customer to remember, so those, in my book, are nixed as well.

Next, choose who will host (display) your created site. There are many companies out there that will host your site for free or for a very small monthly sum, but those hosts will have your site among many others on a generic web page (for example: *www.geocities.com/your-name*). Your website will be a tag on the host parent's site. This may be confusing to your target audience because they will have to surf around the parent site to find you. In my mind, this method is too confusing and inconvenient. If a doctor or patient is looking for me, he or she can find me by using my name in a Web browser. For hosting my site, I compared a few major players, including *www.yahoo.com* and a local company. You can log onto *www.webhostingratings.com*, an independent guide to selecting the right domain Web hosting service for you and your budget. After researching the pros and cons, I felt that a local company would be more accessible and eager to please me. I signed up with *www.smart.net* and pay a $20 monthly fee to host my site. With a domain name in hand and a server to host the site, all you need now is to link your domain name with your site creation and supply it to the host. If you have chosen to have a professional Web designer create your site, supply him with your domain name and host information and get your credit card out. That's it.

Lastly, remember that nothing on your site is written in stone. You can change, add, or delete anything on the site at any time (either by yourself if you have the know-how or through your Web designer/master).

Some men see things as they are and say, "Why?" I dream of things that never were and say, "Why not?"

—*George Bernard Shaw*

CHAPTER 11

Mix It Up:
The Recipe for Success

What Do I Get Out of All This?
What Are Gross Revenue and Net Revenue?

Wouldn't it be just marvelous if we treated a patient, billed the insurance carrier what we determined to be a fair fee, and the insurance company happily cut us a check and mailed it the same day they received it? I hate to burst your bubble, but that Technicolor® dream will never happen. The fee you bill for the services you render is called the *gross revenue*. The insurance company takes that fee, chops it up, purees it, sautés it, and expertly excises a big chunk out of it. That chunk removed is called the *adjustment*. You may also have prenegotiated deals with certain managed care or commercial carriers, or offer a professional courtesy to a carrier and agree to accept less money for promised referral volume or exclusivity. As mentioned earlier in relation to our Medicare discussion, insurance carriers have a secret code phrase for our fees that they call *usual and customary* (U + C). If your fee is more than their U + C, and you can always bet the ranch it is higher, the carrier will trim your fee to what they want to pay. The amount they pay you is called the *net revenue*, also known as gross revenue minus adjustments.

How Much Is It?

Essentially, most if not all therapists establish pricing based on the third party system and government regulations. Different than retail pricing where the shopkeeper takes the wholesale cost and multiplies it by a markup percentage to set his retail price, those of us working in healthcare must consider other issues to establish our pricing.

Medicare Fee Schedule

The Balanced Budget Act (BBA) was signed into law by President Clinton in August 1997. Its multitude of revisions and amendments has had a great effect on how we price our services. For further information on the impact the BBA has made on our healthcare system, log on to *http://www.healthlaw.org/pubs/BBAtoc.html* and *http://www.ebglaw.com/article_326.html*. The government publishes the Medicare Fee Schedule in November of each year in the Federal Register. It is also available to us on the American Physical Therapy Association (APTA) website and *www.PTManager.com*. The Medicare Fee Schedule is also called the Physicians Fee Schedule. It is listing of prices paid to credentialed providers by individual procedural codes called CPT codes. One can learn more about the specifics of each listed code by getting a copy of the CPT Coding manual via the American Medical Association or through *www.amazon.com*.

Basically, the fee schedule is hinged on three factors: (1) a nationally uniform relative value for the specific service, (2) a geographically specific modifier that balances out regional variations, and (3) a nationally uniform conversion factor that is updated annually. To create a fee schedule for one's practice, the therapist must list the services he or she performs, the CPT code for the procedures, the relative value unit factor for each procedure, the geographic modifier for the area, and that year's national conversion factor.

To get your feet wet, and for further information on coding and reimbursement particulars for physical therapists, I advise you to get *The Coding and Payment Guide for the Physical Therapist 2004* (item #4462), published by Ingenix. The spiral bound manual sells for less than $150 with shipping included. It is a bible for new clinicians and business owners, helping them to understand the basics of coding and billing as well as which code to use for what service supplied. APTA has a discount deal program with the publisher so at "check out" time, be sure to look for discount offers. Simply set your browser to *http://www.ingenixonline.com/modules/catalog/catalog_search.asp*.

Once you get comfortable with the whole coding game, you'll need to know what code to bill when you list a given diagnosis. This information can be found in what is called a "crosswalk." Medicare pays only for certain procedures and modalities under each diagnostic (ICD-9) code. For example, for a diagnosis of cervical pain (724.0), Medicare will pay for electrical stimulation (97014), ultrasound (97039), and therapeutic exercise (97110). Interestingly, Medicare will not pay for mechanical traction (97014) or manual techniques (97140), such as joint mobilization, manual traction, or myofascial release. How would you know that? You would think that whatever modality or treatment the therapist provides, as long as it is appropriately documented and effective, would be reimbursed. Not so. Using the crosswalk will give you the edge to plan your treatment and bill effectively. Order item #3219 from Ingenix (*http://www.ingenixonline.com*).

PPO and FFS: Proceed with Caution

When you participate with preferred provider groups, they will often pay you a discounted fee-for-service. Expect a high adjustment rate for such an arrangement. Similarly, commercial, workmen's compensation (WC), and managed care companies will try to trim your gross revenue tree by adjusting off large amounts, leaving you with a net much lower than your gross amount billed.

The Billing Game

Then, the $64,000 question is: Why bill more than the insurance companies pay? The answer is that it is a billing game. If I bill what an insurance company chooses to pay me, it is harder, if not impossible, to ever raise my fees. Since they expect my bills to always be more than what they're willing to fork over, the carrier will, in fact, challenge me to lower my fees. In reality, each insurance company pays me a different amount for the same fees billed. If I charge each one what it will pay me, I'll have 20 different fee schedules.

What's the Goal?

The main goal of any business is to be profitable. One method of increasing profitability is to lower expenses. The other, of course, is to raise earnings. Lowering adjustments is a way of minimizing expenses. How can one lower a predetermined adjustment that an insurer sets? The simple answer is to know your payer mix, as noted in the next section.

The Payer Mix

The payer mix is defined as the group of insurance carriers that you deal with on a regular basis. The mix is usually a combination of commercial, WC, personal injury, and Medicare payers. As you could imagine, some carriers pay more for your services and some pay less. Can you guess who pays the most? Read on….

PIP

Generally, Personal Injury Protection (PIP) insurance carriers pay full or near full fee-for-service. The down side of working with PIP carriers is that oftentimes your bills are scrutinized and questioned, extending your collection time. Since time is money, even though PIP pays the most buck for your bang, waiting two years to get the cash lowers the true value of the money.

Worker's Compensation

WC carriers are likewise slow to pay, but most seem to pay higher than commercial carriers. However, with that said, several slick WC carriers have been working hard looking for ways to pay you less. Remember, the less they pay you, the more they keep in their coffers. For example, if you are a credentialed provider with Cigna HMO (presumably to treat Cigna's commercial population) and they pay you $40 a visit for two modalities and an exercise unit, guess what some WC comp carrier is going to hit you with? You got it: the same $40, even though another carrier like Kemper or Traveler's will pay you fee-for-service to the tune of $120 a visit. There is no way to predict if a WC carrier will contract out its services, but be prepared if it does occur. In this atmosphere of carriers holding onto their dollars increasingly tighter, forcing you to take less is likely to become more prevalent as time goes on.

Commercial Carriers

Commercial carriers such as Blue Cross Blue Shield, including preferred provider groups like Aetna and Prudential, pay a discounted fee-for-service. The magic discount amount is dependent on the area of the country in which you are located and the fee schedule the carrier maintains. By and large, commercial carriers pay better than managed care groups and have no real risk attached.

Managed Care and Preferred Provider Groups

Managed care organizations often are the lowest payers, but promise you exclusive referrals or high volume. Always remember that your fee must exceed your cost or not only won't you realize a profit, but you'll end up with a loss. So in answer to the question in the previous section, juggle your payer mix as best you can to gain an inflow of patient referrals from carriers with high reimbursements and low adjustments, taking into consideration the time necessary to receive payment and extent to which your billing department must chase the money owed. Sometimes lower paying carriers turn around your payments rapidly with electronic billing and make your life easier by not bogging you down with all kinds of supporting documentation or authorization numbers. Speedier payment with fewer hassles may be more profitable in the long run than higher paying carriers that make you wait six months to a year for your money and require all kinds of paper trails before you are paid.

The bottom line still remains, unless you want to work for nothing, always be sure that the money received for service rendered is more than the money it cost you to treat the patient. My only exception to this dictum is if I am cornered into doing a "favor" for a current or potential referral source. Charity issues aside, be careful how altruistic you are in being a "good guy." We all have bills to pay and businesses to run.

Risk If You Do and Risk If You Don't

The payers listed previously all carry some level of risk. What do I mean by that? When you sign a contract that you will accept patients from an insurance carrier for a predetermined fee, you should negotiate that fee to be more than your cost or you just lost your shirt. Insurers are not in the business of losing money. Their goal is to get you to provide services to their membership for the lowest possible price to them. Know your costs to provide the service **prior** to negotiating anything. If you snooze, you lose. Or, if your calculations are incorrect or expenses understated, you could lose.

HMOs, PPOs, IPAs, and Other Abbreviated Players: Who Are They?

HMOs, PPOs, IPAs, and other acronyms are nothing to fear. They are just another group of challenges to tame. Here is a brief rundown of each.

HMOs

HMOs are health maintenance organizations. They were all the rage in the 1980s and '90s, attempting to prevent disease and sickness by offering well care as a primary intervention. The well-known Kaiser-Permanente was the first national HMO and runs on a staff model. That means that pretty much all the medical specialties are housed under one roof or facility and refer within that facility. Their goal is to increase their member's wellness and health while decreasing the individual episodes of care needing professional attention. Some HMOs even own their own hospitals and large multispecialty health and surgi-centers. HMOs were formed to save masses of money by restricting care and determining set referral patterns. They limit patients to using providers that agree to take less revenue for a set standard of service. The system backfired and left many patients unhappy and in no better health to boot. HMOs typically pay poorly in an attempt to hold onto their own revenues. Even increasing volume does not help this equation.

The words "capitation" and "case rate" reimbursements are tied to HMOs. Capitation is a reimbursement mechanism that pays the provider a pre-negotiated monthly sum based on a number multiplied by the current membership in the HMO, for example, $0.70 per 10,000 members, per month. This translates to $7,000/month for all care provided to members of the HMO. However, if it costs you more than $7,000 (very likely), you lose. A case rate pays the provider a given, pre-negotiated sum per patient referred no matter how few or how many times you see Mr. X. As you can plainly guess, both of these reimbursement mechanisms are high risk to the provider and low risk to the insurer. Guess who is laughing all the way to the bank?

PPOs and IPAs

PPOs are preferred provider organizations, the largest of which is currently Blue Cross PPO. It pays to be on their roster. They pay you faster and you lose only a few nickels when you are a provider compared to an outsider. Nearly every doctor belongs to the Blue Cross PPO. It is advantageous as a referral tool as well. By enlisting you are enrolled on their website and printed provider books.

IPAs are independent provider associations that physicians formed to counteract managed care infiltration of their market. They attempted to enroll as many patients as they could and tried to make their own provider networks. IPA specialists accepted less in fees to remain aligned with IPA doctors. There are still a few around, but they are not the market strongholds. Risk is much less to the provider in PPO reimbursement.

How to Tame the Managed Care Man-Eating Beast?

Depending where you set up shop, managed care monsters may be the alpha male or just a nearly extinct breed lurking in the area. To recognize their presence and know their market penetration is the beginning of taming them. It is rare that managed care has not seeped into an area to some extent, but if your location has minimal to no managed care presence, skip this section. If you are like me and realize that managed care is still a pretty big player in the area, listen to a few ways to beat them by joining them. If you have chosen to limit your practice to a self-pay, PIP, and/or WC reimbursement system only, your exposure to managed care may be minimal to none. However, don't be caught off guard. If you snooze, you may get locked out. Many PIP and WC payers are now looking to develop "networks" or "panels." These are insurance company code words for a group of therapists who contractually agree to take less reimbursement or other restrictions of care for the advantage of ensuring exclusivity and volume referrals.

In recent times, managed care administrators have come to learn that the public wants quality, personalized, and convenient care even if they are HMO members. In the 1980s and carly 1990s, managed care seemed to divvy out physical therapy referrals to a faceless, nameless corporate chain who provided an acceptable but low standard of care and patients left unhappy. Today administrators are paying attention to their customers, and managed care is again looking to contract physical therapy services to those of us who offer good, quality, personalized care at competitive rates.

The "C" Word: Don't Even Say It!

The days of capitation (it scares me to even utter the term) are mostly over, but some case-rate payment plans remain to remind us of the horror we lived through in years past. In any event, most, if not all, managed care payers have upped their antes and now pay discounted fee-for-service rates for services provided. Jump on that bandwagon if your managed care presence can *up* your daily visit total without decreasing your margin of profit. That means that with the added managed care referrals you will see from contracting with them, your overhead will not need to increase more than the percentage gain you will realize with the managed care dollars collected. For example, if you need to hire another full-time therapist and technician, which will cost you $75,000 annually, and need more space, which costs you an additional $12,000 a year, in order to treat managed care patients that bring in $65,000 in annual net revenues, you are losing the game. On the other hand, if you have the available space and need only to hire one part-time therapist at a rate of $25,000 a year to accommodate the same increase generated by the new managed care referrals, you have squeezed out an additional $40,000 in profits. Without your managed care contract, someone else in the neighborhood would have taken the $40,000 profit and run to the bank laughing all the way. It is crucial to understand that volume alone does not create more profits. It is the calculated margin that puts you ahead.

If You Can't Beat 'Em, Join 'Em

OK, so if I've convinced you to join them so you can beat them, now you need to know how to join them. How can you join them if you don't even know them? The first step in knowing them is to find them. One way to find them is to open the Yellow Pages and look under the heading "Insurance Companies." Each state's insurance commission maintains a website (see *www. naic. org*). Your state's insurance carriers can be found there.

Knowing how to bill and collect your fees is certainly an important component of developing and running your practice. It's equally important to become a participating or credentialed provider with the insurance plans in your geographic area. Becoming credentialed involves a long paper trail process of application and acceptance by each particular insurance carrier. Once accepted, you are considered a member of that insurance company's "panel," and each provider on the panel is listed in the member's provider directory. Besides the major players like Blue Cross and Medicare, in order to diversify your case mix, you have to investigate what other insurance plans, organizations, and carriers are in your area so you can pursue a contract with them. A. M. Best Company, founded in 1899, is a worldwide insurance-rating and information agency with more than 100 years of history devoted to issuing in-depth reports and financial-strength ratings about insurance organizations. It publishes a database, Best Insurance Reports, and offers the largest listing of insurers in the United States. Using the company's online database, you can easily locate most of the insurance company carriers operating in your locale.

Log on to the A.M. Best Ratings and Analysis page (*http://www3.ambest.com/ratings/advanced.asp?template=*

&*BL=0*) and scroll to the bottom. Where it says "Domicile," highlight "United States," then, click on the particular state you wish to investigate in the next pull down menu. Click "search now" and, *viola*, listed before your eyes is every company in your area. Click the individual company name and contact information will appear. Call the company and ask for provider relations, requesting a provider credentialing packet and a fee schedule. Another way to get more information about carriers in your area is to contact your insurance broker. He or she should be able to supply you with an exact Web address or provide you with a printed version of the insurance carriers in your geographic area. Call every carrier and ask for each one's Provider Relations Department. Sweet-talk every person you speak to and request a provider application packet to become a "credentialed provider" with the group, as well as requesting the individual's name with whom you spoke should you need to contact him or her again. Everyone likes to be remembered. If and when you phone or write again, know their name and use it over and over in the conversation or written correspondence. If you are told that the panel is closed, let them know that you have a large patient base in the area and your referring practitioners are asking why they cannot send you their managed care or preferred provider patients. If that doesn't work, ask for the clerk's supervisor and plead your case. If all else fails, beg. If you are situated in a saturated managed care area, you need the contract more than they need you. Be firm but courteous with them on the phone, making sure you get what you want.

The secret to success is constancy of purpose.

—*Benjamin Disraeli*

CHAPTER 12

The Coding Game

What You Code Is What You Get!

In our line of work, most, if not all, of our revenues come from billing and collecting money due from services rendered to patients. As they say, *where there's a bill there's a way*! The way insurers know what we do and for how long we do it is by two sets of codes: CPT and ICD-9 codes.

CPT Codes

Current Procedural Terminology codes, called CPT codes for short, describe medical or psychiatric procedures performed by physicians and other health providers. The codes were developed by the federal government's Centers for Medicare and Medicaid Services (CMS) to assist in the assignment of reimbursement amounts to providers by Medicare carriers. A growing number of managed care and other insurance companies, however, base their reimbursements on the values established by CMS. Since the early 1970s, CMS has asked the American Medical Association (AMA) to work with physicians and other healthcare providers of every specialty to determine appropriate definitions for the codes and to try to determine accurate reimbursement amounts for each code. The AMA publishes a yearly CPT codebook to advise medical facilities and offices of changes and adjustments in CPT codes and directives on how to properly bill for their specific services. No office should be without this excellent reference. The book may be purchased online through the AMA at *http://www.ama-ssn.org/ama/pub/category/3113.html*. Another option is to get a software program that you can download onto your personal digital assistant. Other companies, such as Medical Coding.Net (*http://www.medical-coding.net/*) offer quick reference guides and cards to make it simple for the practitioner to quickly look up a code. Another excellent method to keep your diagnostic and billing codes handy is by using a reference card put out by Ingenix Corporation specifically for physical therapists. The two card set (ICD-9 and CPT codes) costs about $45 and can be ordered on the Internet by logging onto *http://www.ingenixonline.com/modules/*.

Some insurers do not cover certain procedures. For example, federal insurers like Medicare and Federal Blue Cross do not cover phonophoresis or hot packs. Guess what? Don't bother billing them out even if you perform the procedure or modality because they won't pay you for them.

Over time you'll learn which insurers pay for which CPT code billed. From a legal standpoint, certainly bill what you perform, but do not allow the insurance carrier to underpay you for your hard work. Don't omit billing using a procedural code thinking that the fifteen minutes you spent on electrical stimulation was ancillary to the joint mobilization technique you performed. Get all that is coming to you, including billing for softgoods used in therapy (for example, therabands, splints, bandages, and so on).

When given the choice of billing a code that pays more and one that pays less for the same intervention, be smart. Don't let the insurance carrier laugh all the way to the bank because of your ignorance. For example, you will come to learn that a given insurance carrier reimburses $24 for code 97110 (15-minute unit of therapeutic exercise) and $28 for code 97116 (one 15-minute unit of neuromuscular rehabilitation). Say you are working on sit-to-stand balance and strengthening with a patient. Realistically, you can code the exercise as either 97110 or 97116. Wouldn't you always code the activity for the greater reimbursement rate?

ICD-9 Codes

Another set of codes that determine what condition you are treating is called the ICD-9 code. ICD stands for International Classification of Diseases. The ICD codes are linked by a computerized database to the CPT codes to determine what treatments are payable by Medicare and other insurers per diagnosis. What does that mean to you? It means that you must become a coding expert if you want to get paid for what you did for each patient. In addition, it behooves you to become familiar with what each payer reimburses you per CPT code.

 There's no other way out. To maximize your pay for what you do you must become a walking coding dictionary or have a big code chart on your office wall that indicates which procedure codes to bill for the treatment provided. ICD-9 codes are published by many companies. Medicare and some other carriers have specific CPT codes that may not be billed together on any given visit. These codes are for procedures that generally are not performed on the same visit (for example: 97124 massage and 97140 myofascial release). These are called coding edits. Check *www.cms.HHS.gov/physicians/cciedits/default.asp* to see what CPT codes may be billed simultaneously and which are mutually exclusive. This site allows you to download a spreadsheet listing the edits by CPT code. Click the link to "Medicare Evaluation and Management Services."

In addition, Medicare and some other carriers pay for specific CPT codes per each ICD-9 diagnostic code. You may compose your own "crosswalk," listing which CPT codes are paid per ICD-9 by obtaining a listing directly from your regional Medicare intermediary. Unfortunately, the intermediaries list only individual CPT codes and the ICD-9 codes under which the procedure is covered. A crosswalk with ICD-9 headings and CPT code listings under each diagnostic code is most helpful for accurate billing and clean-claim submission. This is a tedious process to create but well worth the effort. Ingenix publishes and sells laminated quick *cheat sheets* with the most commonly used CPT and ICD-9 codes for physical therapy. The laminated sheets are a cheaper option at about $15 each.

Take Charge! How and What Do You Charge for What You Do?

What's a fee schedule? A fee schedule is a list of the most commonly used modalities and procedures you use, indicating the procedural code (CPT code) and the associated fee for each code. In our field, CPT codes are usually grouped as two separate columns: modalities and procedures. Modalities include "hands-off" techniques like mechanical traction (97012) and electrical stimulation (97016) treatments, and procedures are usually "hands-on" techniques like manual therapy (97140) and therapeutic exercise (97110).

So what are we "schedule-ing"? Well, the fee schedule is used by the billing staff to submit bills and collate payments received. It is also used when negotiating with group payers as proof of what you charge your customers. You will generally adjust your fee schedule on an annual basis for cost-of-living percentage increases and to better maximize your monies received, especially with payers who reimburse as a percentage of what is billed. Usual fee increases hover around 2–3% per year across the board. For an example of a realistic fee schedule, flip to the Appendix.

How to Get Paid for What You Do

It is mind-boggling to think that the process of generating a charge (fee) through finally receiving your due reimbursement takes 17 steps. That's what P.T. Manager.Com's Peter Kovacek calls the Life Cycle of a Claim. These 17 steps must be completely followed or it is doubtful that you'll get what's rightfully coming to you. Take a look at all 17 steps in the Appendix. Understanding the steps the claim goes through will better prepare you for working with your billing staff and directing them in the process of getting paid. A slip-up on any step will delay or defer your reimbursement. I also encourage you to log onto *www.ptmanager.com* and search the site for many other practice-building techniques and formulae.

Get Hip to HIPAA

Privacy and confidentiality are hallmarks of healthcare. Patients put their trust in us to maintain a professional and private environment in which to carry out their needed care. Confidentiality and privacy mean that patients have the full right to control who sees their protected health and personal information. It is our duty to protect this information from others. The Health Insurance Portability and Accountability Act of 1996 (HIPAA) is a federal law that protects a patient's right to have his or her health information kept private, secure, and confidential. Harsh penalties are levied upon those providers who do not uphold this law. Since April 14, 2003, the effects of HIPAA will be evident in any and every medical office, facility, and hospital in the United States.

In your practice, you must uphold the law and protect patient information. Protected health information includes any and all patient medical history and other sensitive data that patients offer us so we can provide appropriate care to them. Sensitive data include the patient's identity, address, age, social security number, and other medical and personal information we ask him or her to provide us. We use the information to plan care for the patients and use specific data for billing purposes. We may use the information when we perform peer-review and quality assurance assessments.

You should always ask yourself prior to looking at potential sensitive information: Do I need to see this information in order to do my job? For example, the receptionist has no need to see the patient's past medical history information and, as such, it should remain confidential from her perspective. The HIPAA law states that the "minimum necessary" information should be shared with others in the office. The concept of "need to know" means that specific information is required for the individual to receive the necessary and appropriate care in the clinic. As healthcare providers, we must all make a reasonable effort to disclose or use only the minimum necessary amount of protected information in order to do our job. We must balance the minimum necessary determinations against our need for information in order to provide quality of care. There is no minimum necessary when it comes to patient treatment. There will still be instances when you will have to access protected health and personal data that you do not need for your specific job. Healthcare providers may disclose to consulting physicians and other providers any and all necessary private information for patient care. Clinicians, however, must be careful about what is disclosed to nonclinician staff about their patients' personal and private information.

To comply with federal regulations, I've outlined the following two rules for my practice:

RULE 1: If someone asks for information about a patient's case, ask why it is needed and disclose only the minimum amount necessary for that person to do his or her job.

RULE 2: As an employee of Esterson & Associates Physical Therapy, part of your job is to help maintain privacy for patients as they undergo treatment with us. It is expected that all staff adhere and comply with HIPAA policies. Employees are encouraged to report privacy violations to the Administrator without any fear of retaliation. Patients also have the right to report violations. If a patient suspects that we are not complying with HIPAA regulations, he or she may file a complaint with the Office of Civil Rights in the U.S. Department of Health and Human Services.

Who is authorized to see protected information? Your entire staff should contribute to the outstanding care you offer. However, that, in itself, does not mean that everyone needs to see health information about each patient. It is common sense to know that staff, under no circumstance, should speak about patients outside the office. In the course of doing your job, you may see patient health information. That information is meant to be available solely for those who require it to perform the indicated care. It is not to be used by any staff member in any way or told to anyone, even if they ask you. The patient is the only one who can authorize staff to divulge private information.

How is patient privacy protected? Patients expect and deserve privacy to the maximum extent we can provide. Keep these pointers in mind:

◆ **Patient care or discussion about patient care should be kept as private as possible by closing doors or drawing curtains to separate the staff and the patient from others, and/or using background music to blur conversations.**

◆ **Always knock or announce yourself before entering a patient's area (door or no door).**

- ◆ Keep patient records locked in a file cabinet, away from the public areas. If charts and records are found unattended or in a public area, the information must be secured and returned to its proper place immediately. Chart sections showing private and confidential data are not to be left in open, clear public view at any time.

- ◆ When a patient is announced/called, do not include any hints or information that would allow others to identify who the patient's physician is, the problem he or she is being treated for, and other identifying data.

- ◆ If others ask staff about another patient's information, politely inform the requester that patient confidentiality law does not allow you to divulge any information about another patient's care, no matter the reason.

- ◆ If possible, begin new patient intakes in a private location, as the environment allows.

- ◆ When a patient chart is in your possession, you are responsible for keeping it secure. Do not leave a chart in areas where others can easily view it. Once you are finished with the chart, return it to its stored/secured location.

- ◆ When and if you have access to electronic patient data, log off the system when you are finished with it.

- ◆ When discarding hard copies of patient information, be sure to shred the paper. Leaving crumpled patient data paper in a trashbin can tempt even the most innocent person and lead to a breach in privacy.

- ◆ It is everyone's responsibility to inform co-workers if you can overhear confidential and private information so that everyone is compliant with the law.

A patient may authorize you to use protected information for purposes other than treatment, payment, or routine operations by giving you written permission to do so. Patients may revoke this authorization at any time in writing. Patients may also ask you to restrict how their medical information is used to carry out treatment, payment, and healthcare operations, although you are not required to comply with their request. In addition to federal law, each state has laws to protect the patient's medical record.

Notice of Privacy Practices

HIPAA requires healthcare providers to have notices telling patients how we will use their information. Esterson & Associates Physical Therapy's Notice of Privacy informs all patients that they have a right to see their own records, make copies, and request amendments in the record. Every new patient receives this notice before receiving care from us. The notice is posted in our waiting room in full view for patients to see and read. We are required to ask patients to acknowledge receiving our Notice of Privacy Practices form. This explains the ways we use patient information and offers the patient the right to view and obtain copies of records and request amendments to the record. In order for a patient to inspect and/or copy protected health information, he or she must complete appropriate forms to request access to or have a protected record copied. HIPAA allows flexibility for a healthcare provider to exercise professional judgment to deny access or provide limited access in special cases where revealing data could be harmful to the patient.

Requested Amendments to the Patient Record

HIPAA allows patients to request amendments to their medical records. You are not required to automatically change anything requested; however, patients must be allowed to make requests and follow a specific protocol to handle the request. You should:

◆ **Respond to the amendment request within 60 days by either accepting or denying the amendment.**
◆ **Inform the patient in writing whether the amendment is accepted or not. It can be denied when the information is in dispute or inaccurate, or when the requested changes are from another facility (for example, X-ray report).**

Electronic Privacy Rules

HIPAA does not specifically address faxing or e-mailing patient information. The law does protect this means of data-sharing under the privacy rule like any other form of healthcare information. The following are two rules Esterson & Associates

Physical Therapy enforces as they apply to patient privacy and electronic media:

- **Faxes: When patient information is faxed, be sure information is sent to a dedicated fax machine, and that you notify the intended recipient when you are sending the information so it can be retrieved immediately. Avoid allowing unattended paper faxes to remain in the fax machine tray for everyone to access. Our fax cover sheet has information about returning improperly addressed faxes and how to dispose of confidential and private information. (See Appendix for a sample of our fax cover sheet.)**
- **E-mail: You can never be sure who has access to a message sent over the Internet. Always check that you have addressed the e-mail to the correct person you intend to read the message. Do not share e-mail addresses or logon codes with other staff members.**

The following demonstrates ways you can protect patient privacy:

1. Close patient room doors/curtains when discussing patient treatments or administering care.
2. Speak softly in semi-private areas when discussing patient information and administering care.
3. Avoid discussions about patients in public areas.
4. Do not leave information on answering machine/voice mail regarding patients or test results.

Potential consequences of breaking HIPAA's rules and regulations can mean either civil or criminal penalty for the staff and the corporation. Civil penalties can result in fines of up to $100 for each violation of the law per person, up to a limit of $25,000 for violating each identical requirement or prohibition. For example, if one staff member discloses the social security numbers of 10 patients, he or she is liable for $100 multiplied by the 10 patients, equaling a $1,000 fine. Criminal penalties for wrongful disclosure can be up to $250,000 and a prison sentence of 10 years.

Being ignorant of the law is never an excuse. Log onto *http://www.hhs.gov/ocr/hipaa* for full details of the law and how to put policies and procedures in place in your practice.

One needs something to believe in, something for which one can have whole-hearted enthusiasm. One needs to feel that one's life has meaning, that one is needed in this world.

—*Hannah Senesh*

CHAPTER 13

Accounting Numbers

How to Keep Afloat in the Sea of Cash: Receivables and Payables

Receivables are monies owed to you. Payables are monies you owe vendors. To track the money that is owed to you, accountants and others *age* your accounts receivable. This means that you may generate income on a Monday, but may not get paid for what you did until three Tuesdays from now. In order to keep things in order, it is important to keep a trail of the money owed from when it was actually generated. This way you know how long it takes to actually receive money in hand for services you performed some time ago. This is called an aging report. The report is a listing by patient or by insurance carrier followed by columns titled 0–30 days, 31–60 days, 61–90 days, and greater than 90 days. Each line has a patient's name and how much is owed on his or her account in each time period. Fact: The longer your money sits out there uncollected, the lower the possibility you will ever collect it. So, it is paramount that you collect your money as fast as possible. Cash is king! Grab it and run!

In recent times with the advent of computer online billing, turnaround time is now days to weeks, as opposed to months to years. Your computer billing program will have an accounts receivable module that tracks your aged receivables. The report is only as good as the person who reads and interprets it. The report can be a method of assessing your billing clerk's performance and to better focus him or her on accounts that need more attention. For those of you who choose to outsource your billing, the company will offer you aged reports to peruse. Read the reports thoroughly and meet with the company to maximize your collections.

Payables are usually the most neglected part of an owner's attention. It is a shame because without our vendors, we would all be up the creek. Our vendors supply us with our goods and keep us stocked appropriately. Not paying them on time is a contradiction in terms. We want our customers to pay us on time so we should return the favor with our vendors.

Note that some vendors offer discounts if you pay the bill in full by an early date. For example, if you pay the invoice in 10 days, the vendor may take 8% off the bill. For example, the company where I purchase my Theraband™ charges me $45 a roll plus shipping. When the invoice arrives, the amount due is $52.50. If I pay within 10 days, I am offered an 8% discount saving me $4.20 on the order. This is a very common way for vendors to encourage you to pay up earlier than later. Like us, money in their pocket now is better than waiting weeks or months to get a bill paid. If you can afford to do so, pay it early and get the discount. You will have a better working relationship with the vendor if you stay in his or her good graces. That way, when one day you need a quick favor for an item you misplaced, the vendor will ship it over in a flash knowing payment will be made *one, two, three*. Many physical therapy vendors call on multiple clinics a day, selling and showing new products. You can gain some valuable marketing tips asking how your peers are faring.

What's a 941 Payment and Other Numbers Your Accountant Will Throw Your Way?

As an employer, you are responsible for paying taxes from your employees' wages along with other taxes like unemployment tax on a monthly, quarterly, or yearly basis. Your accountant will direct you what, when, and how much to fork out. I don't know why, but the accountant always smiles when he or she tells you what you owe. And, you *always* owe!

The most commonly paid tax is the 941. It is the payroll tax that employers pay to the bank after each pay period. Depending on the amount of your payroll, the 941 payment may be due days after the payroll check is cut or monthly. If paid monthly, the 941 is due on the fifteenth of the month for the prior month's payroll withholdings. For example, 941 taxes are due on February 15th for the previous January's total payroll. The employer is responsible for paying double the social security and Medicare withholding (that is, the employee's portion added to the employer's contribution) plus the federal tax withholding for each payroll. The deducted amount on the payroll check is calculated either manually (using tables that the Internal Revenue Service (IRS) will happily send you upon request), by your payroll software program, or by a payroll service. The employer cuts a check made out to the bank for the proper amount and submits it to the bank teller with a voucher that says 941 and the specific quarter it is for. The vouchers are from a voucher book that the IRS sends you when you originally apply for your Tax Identification Number (TIN) (see Chapter 2 to learn about the TIN).

Not all businesses pay the same level of taxes. For example, there is no corporate tax pertaining to LLC and S corporations since the dividends flow directly through to your personal tax bracket and account (refer to Chapter 2 to learn about the various corporate structures).

Besides the 941, here are other taxes that I pay and so will you:

◆ **Form 940** is for the FUTA tax, the Federal Unemployment Tax Act, a fund that employers pay into to cover unemployed individuals. The FUTA rate is .008 of the first $7,000 per employee as long as State Unemployment is paid on time. If not, you are penalized with a higher amount due. This amount is paid for fully by the employer.

◆ **State Withholding** is state tax monies the employer deducts from an employee's payroll check that must be remitted to the state where the business operates. You are required to pay that deducted amount a given number of days after each payroll period, monthly, or quarterly.

◆ **SUTA** is the State Unemployment Tax Act (also known as state unemployment insurance). This tax is paid solely by the employer and is not deducted from the employee's check. State unemployment tax rates fluctuate by state. In Maryland, for example, the SUTA rate is at a minimum 0.003 percent of the first $8,500 per person. SUTA payments are due by the last day of the month for the prior month.

Some taxes vary by the state where you operate your business. The table that follows will give you an overview of the taxes and your responsibilities when paying. Some states have recently accelerated certain tax payment due dates when a company's tax liability is above a given figure. This is, of course, a good way for Uncle Sam to get his hand in your pocket faster and more regularly. Seek guidance and assistance from your trusted accountant to keep you abreast of all tax liability requirements and changes. One word of caution: No matter what your cash status is in a particular month, always have the money available to pay your taxes. It will save you from severe and costly penalties and keep you off the bankruptcy trail or worse.

The breakdown of payroll and other taxes is as follows:

Table 13-1. Payroll and Other Taxes

Tax Type	Company Pays	Employee Pays	Total	Ceiling
Federal Income	None	Variable, see tax table	Depending on salary bracket, 10%, 25%, 28%, 33%, or 35%	Variable, depends on filing status
State Income	None	Variable, see tax table	Varies state to state	Variable, depends on filing status
Social Security	6.2%	6.2%	12.4%	$94,200 gross payroll
Medicare	1.45%	1.45%	2.9%	No ceiling
Federal Unemployment	6.2%	None	6.2% less the State percent	$7,000 payment per employee
State Unemployment	Varies state to state	Varies state to state	Varies state to state	Varies state to state

A word to the wise ain't necessary, it's the stupid ones who need advice.

—*Bill Cosby*

CHAPTER **14**

I Need Help!

How Do I Know How Much Help I'll Need to Start?

Realistically, unless you have provider contracts with payers that will guarantee you business on day one, you will initially be more involved in marketing and personal selling than treating patients. There is no need to hire a full complement of staff before the patients are stampeding through your door. Hiring a well spoken, courteous, assertive individual who is willing to multi-task for a few months as you get the practice rolling is your best bet. He or she can initially act as your front desk person who is willing to assist you in some patient care and office maintenance duties.

As the business owner, you will be forced to wear several hats in the beginning. You will be the marketing professional, office manager, banker, fix-it-person, accounts payable manager, payroll clerk, laundry person, and hold many other jobs. You will eventually delegate many of these jobs to others once you get busier and more involved in treating patients and managing the practice.

What About Employees, Handbooks, and Other Human Resource Resources?

As you get busier, you will need to determine when to hire another therapist, a full-time receptionist, aide, and billing clerk. It would be quite overwhelming to treat 15 patients a day, manage the books, oversee the clerical end, do the laundry, and vacuum the rugs.

Every practitioner is different. You might see 10–15 patients a day and manage running the practice fine. Whatever number is comfortable for you, once the schedule exceeds it, you will need to hire some real staff.

Finding **Sharp** Staff in a Haystack (Try Networking!)

I have **never** been very successful in attracting qualified, competent candidates by advertising in the newspaper classifieds; others may feel differently. Classified advertising usually brings tons of applicants with slim pickings of qualifications. If you must advertise for staff in a classified newspaper, perhaps try to find a community newspaper that tends to serve the area in which your practice is located. Having employees that live close to their place of employment tends to keep them arriving on time (it's hard to get stuck in traffic when you live three blocks from the office) and minimizes the aggravation many others experience on a rainy or snowy day getting stuck in beltway backups and other snarls.

In addition to advertising for staff in the local newspaper's Sunday classifieds, we have some monthly newsmagazines and advertising publications dedicated to physical therapy and other rehabilitation professions. *Advance for Physical Therapists* is probably the most well known monthly publication around. Each monthly print and online issue reports on case study articles, advances in research, reimbursement, political and clinical news, product information, and continuing education opportunities for physical therapists and assistants. At least half of the 150 or so page magazine is dedicated to job opportunity advertisement. The ads are grouped by geographic area and state, making it easy for you to place an ad to attract staff to your "neighborhood." A sharp, one time, small 1″ to 2″ column ad in *Advance* will cost you less than a local city newspaper Sunday classified ad placement plus you will advertise directly to your target market—physical therapists. If you have a logo, include it. It makes the ad more attractive on the page. The advertising department of the magazine is very helpful in designing the ad for you.

Another creative way to advertise for staff therapists is by direct mailing. For a fee (usually about $150), your state chapter of the American Physical Therapy Association sells its membership mailing list in ready-to-use stick-on label format. On your computer, print up an eye-catching, attractive copy to be printed on an oversized postcard advertising your clinic, your philosophy of treatment, and your staffing needs. Brag all you can about how wonderful your practice is and exactly what you, as a boss, are seeking. Two-color printing is more expensive than one color, but the second color makes the card much more attractive. Take your camera-ready copy to Kinko's© or other printing shop for printing. Interested readers will be apt to call you if the location, patient caseload, equipment, and "look and feel" of your place grabs their interest. When I sent out these cards, I received calls from therapists who, prior to receiving the card, were not even looking for a new job. The card piqued their curiosity!

Lastly, there are online classified advertising websites and listservs that directly market physical therapists. Here are a few: *www.ptjobs.com, www.apta.org/bulletin/job_listings*, and others. Set your Web browser to: P.T. Jobs for more sites. It never hurts to advertise for staff using any and every affordable mechanism you can. The above three ways worked for me.

All in all, I have found that the best mode of hiring new staff (professional, supportive, and clerical) is through connections with others—*through the proverbial grapevine*, or networking. A good technician may know another great worker. A crackerjack therapist may have worked with another top-of-the-line therapist who is looking for a new challenge. Inform your staff of your interests or plans to hire new people. They will be your best source for qualified, motivated, and interested candidates. Word of mouth advertising, aimed through the right channels, may bring you more qualified, fitting, and appropriate possibilities, the *sharpest needles* in the haystack!

Eeny, Meeny, Miney, Moe. How to Pick a Winner and Not a **Shmoe?**

The characteristics I deem important for hiring anyone to work in my clinic are the following ones:

◆ **Outstanding customer (patient or referring physician) service**
◆ **Excellent coping skills and ability to deal with stress and frustration (such as patients in pain)**

- ◆ **Excellent communication skills (verbal and written)**
- ◆ **Excellent technical skills**
- ◆ **Attention to detail**

In the interview, I make it clear to the candidate that there are no "trick questions," so they can take time to think about their responses prior to offering their reply. The goal of the interview chat is to clarify for me the applicant's personality, drive, goal-direction, and overall interest.

The most important precursor to hiring qualified and compatible staff is to have a clearly written and concise job description. Describe the job as it really exists, including the interesting and the mundane aspects. When interviewing candidates, let them do the talking. There are many books written on the subject of interviewing. Get a few and read them. Know what you are looking for in each individual job category. For example, a billing clerk requires different personality traits than a staff therapist. If you are like me and value customer service above all, you will want to build a team of people who share the vision of "exceeding each patient's expectations" by making a great first impression and always making the patient feel welcome and at home, visit after visit.

When interviewing the candidates, ask about:

- ◆ **Their recent prior work situation**
- ◆ **The time they went all out for the company and how it was a satisfying experience**
- ◆ **What they feel is their best asset or personality trait**
- ◆ **What they feel they can add to your team**

Do **NOT** ask about age, personal situations, sexual preferences, disabilities, race, or other potentially discriminatory information. This could leave you open to a lawsuit on grounds of discrimination. Do ask all applicants for a list of references, and if you are interested in an applicant, call every one of the provided references. Ask the previous employer about the applicant's dedication and commitment to the past job, timeliness in completing assigned tasks, and whether the applicant was a team player. Ask if that employer would hire the applicant again, and why or why not. The idea of the face-to-face interview is to gain information to assess the skills and qualifications of the candidate. It is not a forum to request information that is discriminatory or would have a discriminatory impact. The following two websites are good references regarding interview questions to ask and those not to get near: *http://216.239.39.104/search?q=cache: fMlOJtmXCDEJ:www.clahs.vt.edu/HTML/faculty/faculty_search/ manuals/questions_to_ask.pdf+what+not+to+ask+at+an+inte rview&hl=en&ie=UTF-8* and *http://www.princeton.edu/hr/poli-cies/employment/224qa.htm.*

Who Will You Relish and Who Will Not Cut the Mustard?

Can you predict who will be a successful worker? Generally, successful workers are ones who are informed of what to do and who have the ability and tools to do the job. They accept responsibility and are self-motivators, team players, and want to please others. Log onto this site: *http://www.schooltocareer.com/ stc/ijs/skills_interview_questions.htm.* It is a website for interviewees to better prepare for interviews with potential employers. Pay particular attention to the sample questions. I find that they are helpful in wording your questions aimed at which assets an individual may have or particular strengths he or she can lend to the company as a whole. Understand that for each job description, a different set of traits may be desirable. Be sure the selected person is the best fit for the job. If at all possible, do not attempt to fit the job to a less qualified or inexperienced person. Read up on interview techniques and how body language and never-ending interviews make for a poor first meeting. I have included a sample of interview "Tricks of the Trade" and questions to pose to your candidates in the Appendix.

The purpose of my interview questions is to evaluate whether the candidate has the specific qualities and skills required for the position at hand. There are generally no wrong or right answers to the questions; instead, I am looking to discover evidence of qualities such as attitudes, initiative, motivation, energy, and maturity in decision making and task execution. My interest in directing specific questions toward the candidate's past experiences is to appreciate the candidate's articulation of a given problem or scenario, what action was taken, and, most importantly, what lesson or concept was learned from the situation.

Now That I've Got 'Em, How Do I Keep 'Em?

One of the toughest jobs we have as practice owners is keeping our key players happy and motivated. Here's how I do it:

◆ **Be a leader and communicate clearly and directly. Don't beat around the bush when you want to get a point across. Staff appreciate directness and honesty.**

◆ **Be a team player and expect staff to be team players too.**

◆ **Give prompt feedback and compliment staff on a job well done. You'll be surprised how much accolades, especially publicly declared, are appreciated.**

◆ **Offer competitive salaries and be especially generous with other perks, as well. A staff lunch, an afternoon off, a birthday cake, and a department store gift certificate in a paycheck envelope for an outstanding week help make staff feel like family.**

◆ **Recognize staff's contributions to your success and make them feel that it is a shared success.**

Your employees are usually your most expensive asset and also your most valuable. Keeping them satisfied and pleased should be your primary goal.

 An employment agreement is a necessary evil of business. The agreement or contract binds your employee to you and you to the employee. It has clear language on what you as the employer promise the employee (for example, salary and benefits) and what the employee promises you, the owner (for example, not to share your business secrets with others). See the Appendix for a sample copy of an employment agreement.

Play by the Rules: The Employee Handbook

All is fair in a game when every player knows the rules. In the real world, many times the owner makes rules during or after a crisis. Staff may arrive late for work or skip a day without prior notification. The billing clerk's computer was "down" so she decided to take a two-hour lunch. The front desk secretary saw that and left a half-hour early too. The staff therapist took a weekend continuing education course and demanded two days off to compensate her for sitting in that boring course over a weekend, and on top of that wants to be paid too! I could go on and on…

Every practice needs an official rulebook (handbook) to spell out word for word the rules of the business game to each and every staff member. The handbook should be a work in progress since new issues always come up that need addressing and new policies must be made as time evolves. It should cover policies of the office as they relate to disciplining staff, time off, benefits, emergency procedures, etc. The handbook sets the tone of the practice, defines the mission and vision of the business, and establishes the company policies, along with maintaining sanity on the job!

From a legal standpoint, always cover yourself: a clearly written handbook will protect the employer from charges of discrimination and unfairness. The last page of the employee handbook should have a tear-out sheet that each employee signs soon after hire. The sheet indicates that the employee has read the handbook and agrees to comply with the contents. Include a statement called "employment at will." This means that you, as the owner, may dismiss an employee for any cause or reason at any time. Other topics in the handbook should include your office dress/uniform standards, drug and alcohol policy, smoking policy, HIPAA Compliance Policies, an equal opportunity statement, and your mission and vision statements. A sample table of contents for an employee handbook is in the Appendix.

I had six honest serving men; they taught me all I knew. Their names were **where** and **what** and **when** and **why** and **how** and **who**.

—*Rudyard Kipling*

CHAPTER 15

Is It Working Yet?

Outcomes: How Will I Know It's Working?

There are many ways to figure out whether you're succeeding in business. In the business world, your success is assessed by performance monitoring. There are many business gurus who preach about different systems to monitor your progress in private enterprise. According to Peter Kovacek, our daily routine of business (he calls it the "rehab business") goes through the following process:

1. Schedule patients
2. Perform evaluations and treatments, documenting all work performed
3. Bill and manage accounts receivable
4. Learn from the results

Kovacek lists key success outcomes for each of these points (see *http://www.ptmanager.com/starting_a_new_therapy_practice. htm*). If your scheduling process meets with success, patients will be pleased with your availability and you will be able to match staff resources with patient demand. As your treatments and documentation paperwork are appropriately executed, referring practitioners refer you more business. When your billing is done correctly and consistently, you are paid in a timely and appropriate fashion. Finally, by analyzing your clinical outcomes (how many visits did it take to reach a given patient's goals), financial outcomes (how much money did you collect this month compared to other months), and your marketing outcomes (how many new referral source contacts did you manage to get business from this month), you will determine your ongoing performance and evaluate your need to adjust your plan based on hard data.

The most concrete and clear analysis of "How am I doing?" is by looking at your financial situation. Kovacek says that professional financial success is evaluated by looking at quality, quantity, reimbursement, and cost control. Quality could be defined as meeting the plan of care, goals, and time frame to achieve the goals as stated in the patient's initial evaluation. Quantity may assess staff achievement on determined productivity standards and compliance issues. Reimbursement success could be a 100% pass rate of pre-billing audits for clean claims submission. Cost control can be deemed successful when soft good supplies are ordered when needed and payroll accountability matches patients' schedules and needs.

 In a more formal fashion, your accountant should review your three basic financial statements with you at least quarterly, if not monthly. The statements are your income (or profit and loss) statement, your balance sheet, and your statement of cash flows. I have included samples of the three statements in the Appendix.

Here is a brief review of each statement:

♦ **Profit and Loss Statement** shows you the amount of money brought in and spent during the given period (usually monthly or quarterly)

♦ **Balance Sheet** shows you how much you own and how much you still owe at a particular period of time (usually at the end of a quarter as well as on the last day of your fiscal year)

♦ **Statement of Cash Flows** analyzes how much money you really have in your bank account to pay all your bills.

Use your financial statements to help you assess your performance. Manage your practice and determine your successes or adjustment requirements by comparing periodic statements as follows:

♦ **Your Profit and Loss Statement can help you estimate this year's totals for patient visits (*sales*, in the business ver-**

nacular) and expenses. Are your expenses increasing more than you expected? Compare today's numbers with last month's numbers. Are you where you thought you would be?

◆ Your Balance Sheet can help you budget your money by determining what you own and what you still owe. Is the time right to buy another large piece of exercise equipment or expand your physical space? Is it affordable right now?

◆ Your Statement of Cash Flows can be used to set financial goals on a month-to-month basis by estimating what your sales and expenses will be this year, month-by-month.

Your Sanity

Take time after you get the business up and rolling to determine how happy you are with your practice and your progress. Are you deriving satisfaction from operating your practice or is it becoming an overwhelming burden? Are you able to sleep at night, or do the daily problems you face every day in your practice prevent you from truly enjoying your success? Take time for yourself. Remember, if you burn out, your practice will suffer. You are the ringmaster. Get smart—Think of yourself for a change and make sure you take time to *smell the roses* before it is too late!

A Final Note

As a practice owner, you are its chief cheerleader and motivator. What drives you should likewise drive the company. You will be spending significant time and dedication in building your practice. Don't burn out early. Take time off when you can afford to, be proud of your accomplishments, and enjoy hearing from others how well you are doing. You will not always meet with success, and you must learn to roll with the punches and see change and possible losses as opportunities for growth. Remember what we said in Chapter 1? The definition of success varies from one individual to another but no one would deny that earning a good living, gaining the respect of others in your community, having more responsibility, and being proud of what you have built are what motivates entrepreneurs to stir up the gumption, courage, and *chutzpa* to make the move from employment for others into ownership and private enterprise for themselves. When profitability and stability become expected, you have left the *start-up phase* of your practice and are about to enter your *growth years*. Best of luck!

The Meaning of Success

To laugh often;

To win the respect of intelligent people and the affection of children;

To earn the appreciation of honest critics and endure the betrayal of false friends;

To appreciate beauty, to find the best in others;

To leave the world a bit better, whether by a healthy child, a garden patch, or a redeemed social condition;

To know even one life has breathed easier because you have lived.

This is to have succeeded.

—*Ralph Waldo Emerson*

Appendices

1. Sample Balance Sheet
2. Sample Income Statement
3. Sample Statement of Cash Flows
4. Sample Pro-forma Budgets
   Year One (Conservative)
   Year Two
5. Sample Business Plan Outline
6. Sample Fee Schedule
7. Sample Physical Therapy Equipment List (New Office)
8. Break-Even Analysis
9. The Life Cycle of Your Claim
10. Interviewing Tricks of the Trade
11. Pre-Employment Reference Check Form
12. Sample Forms
    Payment Policy Form
    Office Encounter Form (Superbill)
    New Patient Registration Form
    Initial Physical Therapy Examination Form
    Medical History Questionnaire
    Patient Sign-In Sheet
    Assignment of Benefits Form
    Fax Cover Sheet
    Physical Therapy Prescription Pad
    Notice of Patient Information Practices
    Release of Records Form
13. Sample Employee Handbook Table of Contents Outline
14. Sample Employment Agreement
15. Resources for Further Information on Private Physical Therapy Practice

16. State Insurance Carrier List Example (State of Maryland)
17. Opening Day Checklist
18. Wise Words Author Listing

Appendix 1
Sample Balance Sheet

Balance Sheet
June 30, 2003

ASSETS

Current Assets		
Regular Checking Account	$ 106,442.23	
Total Current Assets		106,442.23
Property and Equipment		
Furniture and Fixtures	2,500.00	
Equipment	36,290.50	
Accum. Depreciation-Equipment	<25,798.00>	
Total Property and Equipment		12,992.50
Other Assets		
Total Other Assets		0.00
Total Assets	$	119,434.73

LIABILITIES AND CAPITAL

Current Liabilities		
Loans From Shareholder	$ 10,070.00	
Payroll Taxes Payable	31,057.66	
Total Current Liabilities		41,127.66
Long-Term Liabilities		
Total Long-Term Liabilities		0.00
Total Liabilities		41,127.66
Capital		
Retained Earnings	43,606.83	
Dividends Paid	<43,607.00>	
Net Income	78,307.24	
Total Capital		78,307.07
Total Liabilities & Capital	$	119,434.73

Appendix 2
Sample Income Statement

Income Statement
For the Six Months Ending June 30, 2003

	Current Month		Year to Date	
Revenues				
Professional Fees	$ 89,299.86	100.06	$ 406,393.97	100.04
Patient Refunds	<49.50>	<0.06>	<156.16>	<0.04>
Total Revenues	89,250.36	100.00	406,237.81	100.00
Expenses				
Bank Charges	146.22	0.16	210.44	0.05
Billing Expense	7,401.57	8.29	35,269.09	8.68
Charitable Contributions Exp	0.00	0.00	116.00	0.03
Dictation	375.96	0.42	2,459.09	0.61
Employee Benefit Programs Exp	757.96	0.85	2,443.96	0.60
FICA Expense	7,767.58	8.70	13,301.77	3.27
FUTA	0.00	0.00	396.42	0.10
Gifts Expense	0.00	0.00	62.71	0.02
Licenses Expense	0.00	0.00	259.00	0.06
Penalties and Fines Exp	0.00	0.00	3.07	0.00
Other Taxes	0.00	0.00	100.00	0.02
Office Expense	577.72	0.65	3,417.35	0.84
MUIF	0.00	0.00	972.49	0.24
Printing	0.00	0.00	1,546.13	0.38
Professional Development Exp	0.00	0.00	110.95	0.03
Rent or Lease Expense	9,870.00	11.06	20,470.00	5.04
Repairs Expense	734.00	0.82	974.45	0.24
Salaries Expense	155,027.10	173.70	227,369.54	55.97
Supplies	2,223.75	2.49	7,640.93	1.88
Seminars	0.00	0.00	1,850.00	0.46
Security	2,251.00	2.52	2,251.00	0.55
Workman's Compensation	0.00	0.00	803.00	0.20
Telephone Expense	245.50	0.28	2,077.28	0.51
Utilities	1,125.81	1.26	3,825.90	0.94
Total Expenses	188,504.17	211.21	327,930.57	80.72
Net Income	$ <99,253.81>	<111.21>	$ 78,307.24	19.28

Appendix 3

Sample Statement of Cash Flows

Statement of Cash Flow
For the six Months Ended June 30, 2003

	Current Month	Year to Date
Cash Flows from operating activities		
Net Income	$ <99,253.81>	$ 78,307.24
Adjustments to reconcile net income to net cash provided by operating activities		
Payroll Taxes Payable	42,883.59	27,928.31
Total Adjustments	42,883.59	27,928.31
Net Cash provided by Operations	<56,370.22>	106,235.55
Cash Flows from investing activities		
Used For		
Furniture and Fixtures	0.00	<2,500.00>
Equipment	0.00	<8,203.50>
Net cash used in investing	0.00	<10,703.50>
Cash Flows from financing activities		
Proceeds From		
Used For		
Dividends Paid	0.00	<43,607.00>
Net cash used in financing	0.00	<43,607.00>
Net increase <decrease> in cash	$ <56,370.22>	$ 51,925.05
Summary		
Cash Balance at End of Period	$ 106,442.23	$ 106,442.23
Cash Balance at Beg of Period	<162,812.45>	<54,517.18>
Net Increase <Decrease> in Cash	$ <56,370.22>	$ 51,925.05

Appendix 4

Sample Pro-forma Budgets

Year One (Conservative)

Sample New Clinic Pro-Forma Budget—24 Months

Showing Practice Growth, Peak Cumulative Cash Outflow, and Break-Even Point

	1	2	3	4	5	6	7	8	9	10	11	12
(1) Month	1	2	3	4	5	6	7	8	9	10	11	12
(2) Patient visits per month	30	33	36	40	44	48	53	58	64	71	78	86
(3) Income 10% now 90% at end of 90 days	$300	330	363	3,099	3,409	3,750	4,125	4,538	4,991	5,491	6,040	6,644
Expected Ultimate Collection per visit	$100	100	100	100	100	100	100	100	100	100	100	100
Rent			2,200	2,200	2,200	2,200	2,200	2,200	2,200	2,200	2,200	2,200
(4) Therapist Pay	$4,000	4,000	4,000	4,000	4,000	4,000	4,000	4,000	4,000	4,000	4,000	4,000
Equipment Lease	$1,000	1,000	1,000	1,000	1,000	1,000	1,000	1,000	1,000	1,000	1,000	1,000
Utilities	$250	250	250	250	250	250	250	250	250	250	250	250
Supplies	$300	300	300	150	150	150	150	150	150	150	150	150
(5) Insurance	$200	200	200	200	200	200	200	200	200	200	200	200
(6) PT manag'd care network	$200	200	200	200	200	200	200	200	200	200	200	200
Management Fee							100	100	100	250	250	250
(7) Interest		47	94	142	165	187	205	222	235	245	251	254
(8) Loan Repay												
Expense Total	$5,950	5,997	6,044	5,942	5,965	5,987	6,105	6,122	6,135	6,295	6,301	6,304
(9) Net	-$5,650	-5,667	-5,681	-2,842	-2,556	-2,237	-1,980	-1,584	-1,144	-804	-262	340
(10) Cumulative Net	-$5,650	-11,317	-16,999	-19,841	-22,397	-24,634	-26,614	-28,198	-29,342	-30,146	-30,408	-30,068
(11) VARIABLES												
1st Month: # of visits	30											
Ultimate collection / visit	100											
Rate of Growth / month	1.10											

Source: Private Practice Physical Therapy: The How-To Manual, in the Private Practice Section of the manual, © American Physical Therapy Association, 2002.

Year Two

Pro-Forma Budget for a Start-up Practice

24 Months: Showing practice growth, peak cumulative cash outflow, and break-even point

Month	13	14	15	16	18	19	20	21	22	23	24
Patient visits per month	94	104	114	125	138	152	167	183	202	222	244
Income 10% now 90% at end of 90 days	$7,308	$8,039	$8,843	$9,727	$10,700	$11,770	$12,947	$14,241	$15,665	$17,232	$18,955
Expected Ultimate Collection per visit	$100	$100	$100	$100	$100	$100	$100	$100	$100	$100	$100
Rent	$2,200	$2,200	$2,200	$2,200	$2,200	$2,200	$2,200	$2,200	$2,200	$2,200	$2,200
Therapist Pay	$4,000	$4,000	$4,000	$4,386	$4,825	$5,307	$5,838	$6,422	$7,064	$7,770	$8,547
Equipment Lease	$1,000	$1,000	$1,000	$1,000	$1,000	$1,000	$1,000	$1,000	$1,000	$1,000	$1,000
Utilities	$250	$250	$250	$250	$250	$250	$250	$250	$250	$250	$250
Supplies	$150	$150	$150	$150	$150	$150	$150	$150	$150	$150	$150
Insurance	$200	$200	$200	$200	$200	$200	$200	$200	$200	$200	$200
Network	$200	$200	$200	$200	$200	$200	$200	$200	$200	$200	$200
Management Fee	$250	$504	$751	$1,039	$1,157	$1,379	$1,577	$1,819	$2,073	$2,358	$2,652
Interest	$251	$234	$213	$187	$160	$129	$94	$55	$12	$0	$0
Loan Repay	$1,000	$1,000	$1,000	$1,000	$1,000	$1,000	$1,000	$1,000	$1,000	$1,000	$1,000
Expense Total	$6,301	$6,538	$6,764	$7,413	$7,942	$8,615	$9,309	$10,096	$10,949	$11,928	$12,999
Net	$1,007	$1,493	$2,066	$2,295	$2,734	$3,125	$3,602	$4,104	$4,669	$5,286	$5,968
Cumulative net	-$29,061	-$27,568	-$25,502	-$23,207	-20,473	-$17,348	-13,746	-$9,642	-$4,973	$312	$6,280

Footnotes:
(1) The expected patient visits per month are projected at a very conservative level. The formula increases the visits monthly by 10%.
(2) Income is projected assuming that about 10% will be collected immediately from patients for co-payments, deductibles, and co-insurance.
(3) The amount of income ultimately expected from each visit must be carefully calculated with attention paid to practice patterns including number of procedures per visit, managed care contracts and patient/client mix. The $100 figure used here is based on past experience in the same locale.
(4) The gross amount expected to be paid out to physical therapists should be paid to patient volume, as clinic gets busier.
(5) Insurance costs include Professional Liability, General Liability, and any disability policies that will be payable to the practice in the case of a loss.
(6) If the practice is to participate in a provider network, the costs must be included.
(7) Interest must be paid on all loans and in this case is tied to "cumulative net."
(8) A loan repayment plan was originally incorporated in this model, but later deleted. Owner starts repaying loan out of "net" starting month 12 on this budget.
(9) Revenue minus expenses in a particular month.
(10) Cumulative Net is useful for calculating the amount of loan needed to get through the projected period. The model predicts maximum debt load of $30,408 in month. By manipulating the variables, this could change.
(11) The last 3 lines are 3 important variables. The spreadsheet incorporates these into the formulas, to calculate the results of different growth scenarios.

Source: Private Practice Physical Therapy: The How-To Manual, in the Private Practice Section of the manual, © American Physical Therapy Association, 2002.

Appendix 5
Sample Business Plan Outline

I. Table of Contents
Lists what is found in the Business Plan document.

II. Executive Summary
This section summarizes the meat and potatoes of the Business Plan. Even though the Executive Summary is located in the early portion of the Business Plan document itself, it is written after all the other sections are completed. It is one to two pages long with a paragraph dedicated to each of the sections of the Plan. Finally, a paragraph or two listing the capital requirements of the practice and the return on investment is included. This section is very important because oftentimes it is the only section a busy banker or investor will peruse. To catch their attention, colorful graphs and pie charts are recommended here.

II. Market and Industry Analysis
This section discusses the market need for your practice. Who are your referral sources? Who are your potential customers (referring practitioners and patients)? What other ways can you bring customers through your doors? What managed care or other network potential groups can you enlist? This section requires a significant amount of market research on your part. You must project your guesstimated number of patients in order to come up with your potential sales revenue. The bottom line—how much will you make in a given period and when will the lender see his money back with interest? No one expects you to know exactly how many patients you will drag through your doors in a given period, but you must make fairly accurate estimates from assumptions you come up with and from information you can glean from others.

IV. Business Description

This section clearly and fully explains your practice, the niche you want to develop, and/or the service you wish to sell. Are you a specialist in orthopedic care, sports medicine, myofascial release, or women's health? Describe your service and explain fully why your market wants and needs it. Remember that your market consists of both referring practitioners (you are selling your expertise and service to them) and your patients (who are the end users of your care). Brag a little. Tell the reader why your practice is better than others in the area. This section also includes how the company is organized (a corporation, sole proprietorship, partnership, limited liability corporation, etc.), if stock was issued, who has invested money, and how much was put in. Realize that if you are seeking capital, this section will be carefully and closely analyzed by the potential investor. Keep it clear and honest.

V. The Competition

Who are the major players in the local market? Who are your direct competitors—other practices, hospital outpatient clinics, rehabilitation centers, home care agencies? Show that you know exactly with whom you are competing. Discuss what you believe are the competition's strengths, weaknesses, and penetration of the available market. End this section with what you will do to draw the market to you.

VI. Marketing Strategy

Here, explain how you will let your target audience (referring practitioners, potential patients, health plans, referral coordinators, among others) know who and where you are. How will they know you're in business? What's your marketing approach? Billboard advertising? Brochures? Printed Rolodex® cards? Bagel breakfasts delivered with a prescription card attached? In other words, how will you get the word out that you are "at their service"?

VII. Operations Plan

This section is generally dedicated to describing the logistics of a production business. As a service business, this section will be short for you. You are simply selling yourself and your talents. Discuss how many productive hours per week you will spend, that

is, how many hours a week will you be generating income by seeing patients and how many hours will you be doing administrative
tasks? When will the practice be open? What special evaluations
or treatments will pay you better than others and how many do
you assume you'll do in a given period?

VIII. The Management Team
In this section, boast why you and your team are the best at what you
do. Don't be shy. Tell everyone what your qualifications are and how
determined you are to make this practice work well. Also, add in who
you will need during the early years of growth and why such a person
will be beneficial to the practice. The investor wants to be confident
that his money is going to the right person. Who is that right person?
Yup, the one who makes the money back fast with a nice gravy of
interest on top. The investor is also looking for how good your management and advisory team is (your CPA, lawyer, etc.).

IX. Capital Needs
Up to this point, you've discussed the basics of the newly formed
practice. In this section you'll identify the initial cash outlay and
how much more money you'll need in the future based on your
sales (number of patient visits) and operations (expenses, bills,
adjustments to income, etc.) projections. The bottom line is that
the investor wants to know how much money you need, how much
he or she can expect to make in the deal, and how long until there
are rewards. This is where a break-even analysis will show when
the investor can expect to see a profit on his or her investment.
Pro-forma statements, three accounting reports that your accountant will help you draw up based on your projections of number of visits and anticipated expenses, are included in this section
as well. The three accounting reports are as follows:
  • Pro-forma Balance Sheet: A prediction of what you own (your
    assets) compared to what you owe (your liabilities). It helps the
    investor see whether he or she can use your assets to pay off
    what you owe if you run into trouble.
  • Pro-forma Income Statement: A one-year assumption of how
    much money you'll make compared to how much you'll spend
    over the year. It gives a picture of how much you expect to actu-
    ally earn.

- Pro-forma Statement of Cash Flows: A report that realistically shows what and when you expect to receive money earned over a three-year period (one year month-by-month, and the following two years annually), keeping in mind that you receive money some time after you earn it (insurance companies pay you after you actually see the patient). This statement realizes that there is a time lag between the time you earn the money and the time you receive the money, so it ensures that you won't run out of money to pay your expenses.

X. Appendices

Include necessary charts, office design layout, perhaps specialized (impressive) equipment diagrams, and professional resumes to show the investor that you have supportive documentation for your statements in the sections above and that you are worthy of attention and money.

Appendix 6
Sample Fee Schedule*

*The following is a suggested sample fee schedule and is no way intended to represent price fixing or fee setting.

EXAMINATIONS	CPT CODE	FEE
Initial PT Evaluation	97001	$100
Re-evaluation	97002	$75

PROCEDURES		
ADL Training	97535	$55
Iontophoresis	97033	$50
Pneumatic Compression	97016	$39
Manual Therapy Techniques	97140	$50
Massage	97124	$39
Neuromuscular Reeducation	97112	$55
Therapeutic Exercise	97110	$39
Ultrasound	97035	$39
Gait Training	97116	$39

MODALITIES		
Cryotherapy/Hot Packs	97010	$25
Electric Stimulation	97014	$39
Mechanical Traction	97012	$39
Paraffin Bath	97018	$39
Whirlpool/Hydrotherapy	97022	$44
Aquatic Therapy	97113	$40

TESTS/MEASUREMENTS		
Isokinetic Testing	97750	$100
ROM Measurements	95852	$55
Manual Muscle Tests	95832	$55

TESTS/MEASUREMENTS (continued)	CPT CODE	FEE
Ergonomic Analysis	97799	$150
Biofeedback Training	90901	$50

MISCELLANEOUS

	CPT CODE	FEE
Wound Debridement	11041	$55
Orthotic Training	97112	$39
TENS Electrode Training	64550	$44
Group Exercise Therapy	97703	$55
Unlisted Modality	97039	$39

Appendix 7

Sample Physical Therapy Equipment List (New Office)

ITEM	SIZE/AMT	PRICE EACH	PRICE TOTAL
Exam tables	4	$200	$800
Exam room stools	6	$80	$480
Traction table (hi/lo)	1	$5000	$5000
Ultrasound machine	2	$1250	$2500
Electrical stimulation machine	3	$1200	$3600
Treadmill	1	$3000	$3000
Bike (recumbent)	1	$2500	$2500
Cable column (Biodex®)	1	$3500	$3500
Upper body cycle	1	$2500	$2500
Hydrocollator and packs	1 large	$2000	$2000
Freezer and packs	1	$1500	$1500
Telephone system	1 (4 ext's)	$3000	$3000
Washer/Dryer	1 each	$700	$700
Total gym exerciser	1	$1500	$1500
Cybex NORM (used)	1	$8000	$8000
Evaluation tools (soft goods)	Varied	$500	$500
Start-up printed materials	Varied	$1000	$1000
Basic office supplies	Varied	$500	$500
Waiting room chairs (used)	8	$80	$640
Office chairs (wheeled)	3	$50	$150
File cabinet (used)	1	$200	$200
Miscellaneous	Varied	$1000	$1000
TOTAL			**$44,570**

Including $1875 for one month's rent (for a 1500 square foot clinic @ $15/sq ft), the total *ballpark* figure to open this well-equipped startup practice (excluding salaries) is less than $50,000.

Appendix 8
Break-Even Analysis

GRAPHIC PRESENTATION

Here's how to draw your graph:

1. Set your axes by recording your sales volume (number of patient visits) along the horizontal (X) axis. This axis should extend to the maximum level of sales. Both total revenues (sales) and total costs (fixed costs + variable costs, which are all your expenses to run your practice) are recorded on the vertical (Y) axis.
2. Plot the total revenue line starting at zero activity level. For every patient visit (sale), total revenue will increase by your cost per visit fee. Note that the revenue line is assumed to be linear (see assumptions above).
3. Plot the total fixed costs using a horizontal line because these costs do not fluctuate with the volume of patient visits.
4. On the graph, the amount of the variable cost can be derived from the difference between the total cost and the fixed cost lines at each level of activity.
5. Determine the break-even point from the intersection between the total cost line and the total revenue line. The break-even point in dollars is found by drawing a horizontal line from the break-even point to the Y-axis. The break-even point in patient visits is obtained by drawing a vertical line from the break-even point to the X-axis. At this sales level (patient visit level), the business will cover all costs but make no profit.

In addition to identifying the break-even point, the break-even analysis graph shows both the net income and the net loss areas. The amount of income or loss at each level of patient visits (sales) can be derived from the total sales and total cost lines.

The following illustrates the components of the break-even graph:

Break-Even Graph Components

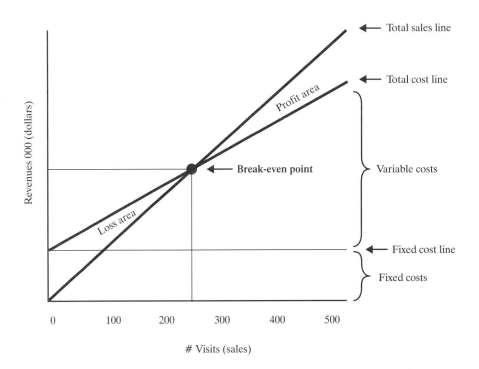

Appendix 9
The Life Cycle of Your Claim

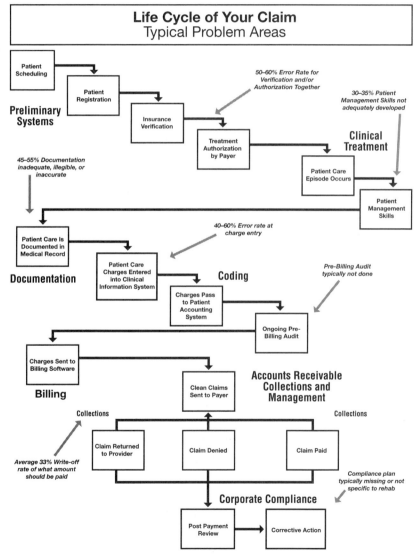

Life Cycle of Your Claim
Typical Problem Areas

Patient Scheduling

Patient Registration

Preliminary Systems

Insurance Verification

Treatment Authorization by Payer

50–60% Error Rate for Verification and/or Authorization Together

30–35% Patient Management Skills not adequately developed

Clinical Treatment

Patient Care Episode Occurs

Patient Management Skills

45–55% Documentation inadequate, illegible, or inaccurate

Patient Care Is Documented in Medical Record

Documentation

Patient Care Charges Entered into Clinical Information System

Coding

40–60% Error rate at charge entry

Charges Pass to Patient Accounting System

Pre-Billing Audit typically not done

Ongoing Pre-Billing Audit

Charges Sent to Billing Software

Billing

Clean Claims Sent to Payer

Accounts Receivable Collections and Management

Collections

Collections

Claim Returned to Provider

Claim Denied

Claim Paid

Average 33% Write-off rate of what amount should be paid

Compliance plan typically missing or not specific to rehab

Corporate Compliance

Post Payment Review

Corrective Action

Source: © 1998 Kovacek Management Services, Inc. and CBL-Solutions, Inc. Reprinted with permission.

Appendix 10
Interviewing Tricks of the Trade

I control the flow and direction of an interview by asking specific questions to probe the candidate in the following areas that I have identified and defined below (with multiple variations and adjustments from years of self-employment experience):

- *Adaptability* is the ability to be flexible in different scenarios. You have probably had the experience of working hard on a project and then being told you must change your priorities. How did you handle that?
- *Administrative interest* is the desire to maintain records and data. What part of your work has given you the greatest feeling of achievement and satisfaction? What part is the most frustrating or unsatisfying?
- *Analysis* allows you to identify and detail ideas and thoughts into useful concepts and direction. Have you ever recognized a problem or an opportunity before anyone else?
- *Control* is a way of self-managing a scheme of things in a focused way. Describe procedures that you have used to keep track of things that require your attention.
- *Decision making* is the ability to choose between different variables. Describe a work-related problem you had to face recently. What method did you use to deal with it?
- *Delegation* is the ability to divide and share control with others. Are you comfortable with allowing someone else to do work that will represent you?
- *Initiative* is a trait of resourcefulness, of being enterprising and inventive. Give me examples of when you went "beyond the call of duty" in accomplishing a work-related project.
- *Integrity* is honesty and reliability in the job and with others. Give me an example of when you had to "bend the rules" in order to get something done.

- *Leadership* is a charisma to direct and manage others. Do you enjoy being a leader? What is the most appealing factor in being a leader? What is the least appealing?
- *Planning* is the ability to project thoughts and ideas toward a goal. How do you plan and prioritize your work week?
- *Verbal communication* is the ability to express yourself verbally in a clear and tactful way. Do you consider yourself direct and to the point or a more detail-oriented communicator?
- *Written communication* is the ability to express yourself clearly and concisely in written format. What is the most difficult writing assignment you have done recently?

Appendix 11
Pre-Employment Reference Check Form

Applicant's name: _____

Date: _____ Telephone: _____

Supervisor's name: _____ Title held: _____

Information supplied by: _____ Title: _____

Employment dates: _____ Position: _____

How long was he/she in the position? _____

What were his/her duties? _____

How would you rate the quality of his/her work? _____

Did he/she get along with others? _____ Peers? _____
Supervisors? _____ Subordinates? _____

Were there any problems with excessive absences/lateness? _____

Was he/she dependable? _____

Does he/she have any physical/mental handicaps that would prevent
him/her from performing assigned duties? _____

Why did he/she leave the job? _____

Would you re-hire/re-employ him/her? _____

Would you recommend him/her for a position as a _____?

Why yes/not? _____

Completed by: _____ Date: _____

Appendix 12
Sample Forms

Payment Policy Form

_____ PRIMARY INSURANCE—We will bill your primary insurance as a courtesy to you. We assume payment of **insurance** benefits is **not forthcoming on charges older than** 60 days. **Charges outstanding for more than sixty days will be due in full from you regardless of the type of insurance involved**. Any remaining balance after your co-pay and your primary coverage has been paid, including items classified as "above usual and customary," is due from you upon receipt of the explanation of benefits from your primary insurance carrier. You will be responsible for any item not paid in full by your insurance carrier. Prior to beginning treatment, we will verify your insurance benefits. While we will take all reasonable action to provide accurate therapy benefit information for your specific plan, be aware that verification of benefits is not a guarantee of payment from your insurance carrier. Secondary insurance will be your responsibility to file and collect.

_____ **MEDICARE**—We will bill Medicare for you. In most cases, Medicare will pay 80% of allowable charges. We will bill your secondary insurance for you, if you have one, or the balance will be billed to you.

_____ **SELF PAY**—Please pay the balance in full at the time of service or upon the receipt of a monthly statement or notice. In the event you are unable to pay the balance in full, we are willing to make reasonable payment arrangements. Please be advised that _Anyone's Physical Therapy Group_ is not a credit grantor, and therefore, failure to maintain these arrangements may result in the placement of your account with a collection agency or attorney for collection. Credit cards (Mastercard and Visa) are accepted for payment on account.

_____ **WORKERS' COMP**—We will bill your Workers' Comp carrier for your charges. Please note that you will remain financially responsible for all of your charges if your carrier denies coverage.

_____ **LEGAL SUIT**—We will accept a legal letter of protection if you meet each of the following criteria:

1. Do not qualify for benefits under any insurance policy (medical or auto), and
2. Are indigent and cannot pay for charges due using cash or credit card, and
3. Are awaiting settlement and subsequent payment of damages from a related legal case, and
4. Return our lien, signed by both you and your attorney.

Prior to your settlement, payment on your account will not be required unless your charges remain outstanding for more than 90 days from the date of last treatment. Upon settlement of your legal case, your balance in full is due within 30 days. Please be aware that you will remain financially responsible for services rendered regardless of the payment option selected above. In the event your account becomes delinquent and is therefore in default of payment, the patient, legal guardian, or admitting parent will be responsible for the principal amount owing, and all reasonable costs associated with the collection of this debt, including, but not limited to, collection service fees, attorney's fees, and all court costs and additional legal expenses associated with the recovery of this debt. We reserve the right to charge interest on balances over 30 days old, charge returned check fees as allowed by state law, and charge a no-show fee for missed appointments when adequate notice of cancellation is not provided. Thank you for allowing us the opportunity to serve you. If you have any questions about the above information or any uncertainty regarding your insurance coverage, please ask for our assistance. Kindly sign and date this document to indicate that you understand and agree to the terms of this payment policy.

CANCELLATION POLICY: To maintain appointment times available for all of our patients, there is a charge of $30.00, *BILLED TO THE PATIENT*, for each instance a patient does not show for a scheduled appointment or does not give at least 24-hour cancellation notice.

☐ Checking this box indicates that the formal office **HIPAA policy and procedures** have been explained to the above-noted patient and that a copy of the policy was provided to the patient.

Assignment of benefits/authorization to release medical information/consent to treatment: I hereby assign all medical benefits to which I am entitled to Anyone's Physical Therapy, P.A. in the event they file insurance on my behalf, I understand that I am financially responsible for all charges whether or not paid by said insurance. In the event my account becomes delinquent and is there in default of payment, I accept responsibility for the principal amount owing as well as all reasonable costs associated with the collection of this debt. This includes but is not limited to collection service fees, attorney's fees, and all court costs and additional legal fees associated with the recovery of this debt. Interest may be charged at a rate of 1.5% per month (12% annually) for unpaid balances over 30 days old. I hereby authorize said assignee to release all information necessary to secure the payment of said benefits. A copy of this assignment shall be considered as effective and valid as the original. I do hereby consent to such treatment by the authorized personnel of Anyone's Physical Therapy, P.A. as may be dictated by prudent medical practice by my illness, injury, or condition. This consent is intended as a waiver of liability for such treatment excepting acts of negligence.

AUTHORIZED SIGNATURE   DATE

Office Encounter Form (Superbill)

ANYONE'S PHYSICAL THERAPY GROUP

ICD-9: _____

Physician's Name _____

PATIENT NAME _____

Insurance _____

DIAGNOSIS _____

EVALUATION & TESTING
[ ] 97001   Initial Evaluation

DATE _____

[ ] 97002   Re-evaluation

_____

PROCEDURE

_____

[ ] 97535   ADL ×___ units

_____

[ ] 97034   Contrast Bach ×___ units

_____

[ ] 97032   Elec. Stim. Attended ×___ units

_____

[ ] 97116   Gait Training ×___ units

_____

[ ] 95851   Goniometry

_____

[ ] 97033   Iontophoresis ×___ units

_____

[ ] 97016   Pneumatic Compression

_____

[ ] 97530   Therapeutic Activities

_____

[ ] 97140   Manual Therapy Techniques ×___ units

_____

Joint Mobilization

_____

Manual Traction

Myofascial Release

[ ] 97124   Massage ×___ units

[ ] 95831   Muscle Testing

[ ] 97112   Neuromusc. Re-education

[ ] 97750   Physical Performance Test

[ ] 97520   Prosthetic/Orthotics Check ×___ units

[ ] 97110   Therapeutic Exercises ×___ units

[ ] 97035   Ultrasound ×x___ units

[ ] 97542   Wheelchair Management ×___ units

[ ] 97564   Each additional hour

MODALITIES
[ ] 97113   Aquatic ×___ units

[ ] 97010   Cryotherapy/Hot Packs

[ ] 97014   Elec. Stim. Unattended

[ ] 97012   Mechanical Traction

[ ] 97018   Paraflin Bath

[ ] 97022   Whirlpool

MISCELLANEOUS
[ ] 99071   Educational Supplies

[ ] 97703   Orthotics Check ×___ units

[ ] 97504   Orthotics Training/Fitting ×___ units

[ ] 99002   Orthotics/Foot

[ ] 97799   PCE

[ ] A4454   Taping

REHABILITATION POTENTIAL
Initial + Re-evaluation visit only
[ ] Good   [ ] Fair   [ ] Poor

WOUND CARE/DEBRIDEMENT
[ ] 11040   Skin partial thickness

[ ] 11041   Skin full thickness

[ ] 11042   Skin & subcutaneous tissue

[ ]   Supplies _____

_____   _____   _____ TOTAL
THERAPIST SIGNATURE   LICENSE #

[ ] No Show   [ ] Cancel

New Patient Registration Form

PATIENT INFORMATION							
LAST NAME	FIRST	MI	DATE OF BIRTH / /	AGE	SOCIAL SECURITY NUMBER		SEX
HOME ADDRESS		CITY	STATE	ZIP CODE		HOME PHONE	
MARITAL STATUS SINGLE [ ] MARRIED [ ] OTHER [ ]	HAVE YOU EVER RECEIVED PHYSICAL THERAPY IN THE PAST? IF SO, WHERE?						
EMPLOYMENT STATUS EMPLOYED ( ) FULL TIME STUDENT ( ) PART TIME STUDENT ( ) N/A( )			EMPLOYER NAME/SCHOOL NAME			TITLE/POSITION	
WORK ADDRESS		CITY	STATE	ZIP CODE		WORK PHONE	

EMERGENCY CONTACT, LEGAL GUARDIAN, INSURED INFORMATION				
LAST NAME	FIRST		MI	HOME PHONE
ADDRESS		STATE		ZIP CODE
EMPLOYER		WORK PHONE		

REFERRING PHYSICIAN INFORMATION				
LAST NAME	FIRST		MI	UPIN #
ADDRESS		TEL #		FAX #

REASON FOR TODAY'S VISIT	
PLEASE DESCRIBE INJURY / ACCIDENT / ILLNESS: (CIRCLE ONE)	
TYPE OF ACCIDENT	DATE

PRIMARY INSURANCE COMPANY INFORMATION					
PRIMARY INSURANCE COMPANY NAME		EFFECTIVE DATE	IDENTIFICATION NUMBER		GROUP NUMBER
ADDRESS	CITY	STATE	ZIP CODE	PHONE	
POLICYHOLDER (if other than patient)	SS#		RELATIONSHIP	DATE OF BIRTH	
(CIRCLE ONE) SCRIPT / REFERRAL	AUTH #		AUTH DATE	EXP. DATE	
COPAY / COINSURANCE		DEDUC. AMT.	MET ☐ YES ☐ NO	MAX # VISITS	
ADJ / CASEWORKER		TEL #		FAX #	

SECONDARY INSURANCE COMPANY INFORMATION					
SECONDARY INSURANCE COMPANY NAME		EFFECTIVE DATE	IDENTIFICATION NUMBER		GROUP NUMBER
ADDRESS	CITY	STATE	ZIP CODE	PHONE	
POLICYHOLDER (if other than patient)	SS#		RELATIONSHIP	DATE OF BIRTH	
(CIRCLE ONE) SCRIPT / REFERRAL	AUTH #		AUTH DATE	EXP. DATE	
COPAY / COINSURANCE		DEDUC. AMT.	MET ☐ YES ☐ NO	MAX # VISITS	
ADJ / CASEWORKER		TEL #		FAX #	
INSURANCE REP.		DATE OF VERIFICATION		VERIFIED BY	

Initial Physical Therapy Examination Form

ESTERSON & ASSOCIATES PHYSICAL THERAPY
INITIAL EXAMINATION FORM

Patient Name: _____ Date: _____ MD/PT Dx: _____

Primary Physician: _____ Specialist Physician: _____

Age: _____ Occupation/Work Activites: _____

Next Referring MD Visit: _____ **Contraindications/Pre** _____

Onset Date: _____ History of Current Diagnosis: _____

_____

_____

Subjective Complaints: _____

☐ Pain _____   ☐ Weakness   ☐ Altered Gait   ☐ Decreased Functional Mobility
☐ Decreased ROM   ☐ Altered Balance   ☐ ADL Difficulty   ☐ Altered Stair Negotiation
☐ Stiffness   ☐ Swelling   ☐ Requires Assistive Device ☐ Disturbed Sleep

☐ PMH Form Completed   ☐ Medications Listed   ☐ Diagnostic Tests _____

BP: / HR: Resp: _____

Prior Level of Function: ☐ No limitations ☐ Limitations: _____

Current Level of Function: ☐ No limitations ☐ Limitations: _____

Posture: ☐ Kyphosis _____ ☐ Lordosis _____ ☐ Scoliosis _____ ☐ Lateral Shift _____
☐ Iliac Crest Height _____ ☐ PSIS _____ ☐ ASIS _____ ☐ Other _____

Gait: ☐ Assistive Device _____ Pattern: _____

Heel Toe Walk   ☐ yes   ☐ no _____

Palpation ☐ Tender   ☐ Tight   ☐ Increased Tone/Spasm   ☐ Spasticity   ☐ Spongy   ☐+ Jump Sign

Upper Quarter: _____

Lower Quarter: _____

ROM:_____

Strength: Left _____# Right _____# (Dynamometer Level 1 2 3 4 5)

Sensation: ☐ Intact ☐ Diminished_____   ☐ Light Touch ☐ 2 Point Discrimination
Proprioception: ☐ Intact ☐ Diminished _____   Kinesthesia: ☐ Intact ☐ Diminished_____
Balance: Static: _____ Dynamic: _____ Functional Reach: F _____L ____ R _____

DTRs:	Left	Right
Biceps (C5)	_____	_____
Brachioradialis (C6)	_____	_____
Triceps (C7)	_____	_____
Quadriceps (L4)	_____	_____
Medial Hamstring (L5)	_____	_____
Gastrocnemius (S1)	_____	_____

Edema: _____
| | ☐ +1 | ☐ +2 | ☐ +3 |

Joint: _____   R _____ L _____
_____ R _____ L _____
_____ R _____ L _____
Skin: _____ Pulses: _____

R ___ L ___ shoulder elevators (C4)   R ___ L ___ hip flexors (L1-2)
R ___ L ___ shoulder abductors (C5)   R ___ L ___ knee extensors (L3)
R ___ L ___ elbow flexors/wrist extensors (C6)   R ___ L ___ ankle (L4)
R ___ L ___ elbow extensors/wrist flexors (C7)   R ___ L ___ great toe extensors (L5)
R ___ L ___ thumb extensors (C8)   R ___ L ___ ankle PF, knee flexors, hip extensors (S1)
R ___ L ___ hand intrinsics (T1)   R ___ L ___ toe and knee flexors (S2)
R ___ L ___ shoulder ER   ___ trunk extension
R ___ L ___ shoulder IR   ___ abdominals

Initial Physical Therapy Examination Form (continued)

ESTERSON & ASSOCIATES PHYSICAL THERAPY
INITIAL EXAMINATION FORM

Patient Name: _____

Special Tests (+/-):

R __ L __ Cervical Quadrant	R __ L __ Thoracic Slump (Dural stretch)
R __ L __ Cervical Compression/Distraction	R __ L __ Lumbar Slump
R __ L __ Roo's (TOS)	R __ L __ SLR R _____degrees L _____ degrees
R __ L __ Adson	R __ L __ Prone Knee Bend (U/L L2 3 nerve; B/L instability)
R __ L __ Load and Shift/Relocation (A/P Instability)	R __ L __ Lumbar Quadrant
R __ L __ Sulcus Sign (Inferior Instability)	R __ L __ Leg Lengths _____
R __ L __ Hawkins-Kennedy (Impingement)	R __ L __ Trendelenburg
R __ L __ Neer (Impingement)	R __ L __ Gillet Sacral Fixation
R __ L __ Speed's	R __ L __ Thomas
R __ L __ Yergason's	R __ L __ Ober
R __ L __ Empty Can	R __ L __ Faber
R __ L __ Lift Off	R __ L __ Piriformis FAIR
R __ L __ Clunk Test (Labral Lesion)	R __ L __ Anterior/Posterior Drawer
R __ L __ Lachman's	R __ L __ Upper Limb Tension
R __ L __ Elbow Ligamentous Instability	R __ L __ Varus/Valgus Stress _____
R __ L __ Apley Compression/Distraction	R __ L __ Plica
R __ L __ Lateral Epicondylitis I II	R __ L __ Clarke's Sign (Patellar Grind)
R __ L __ Elbow Flexion Test (Ulnar nerve)	R __ L __ Q-Angle _____ degrees
R __ L __ Pinch Grip (Median n.)	R __ L __ Noble Compression (ITB)
R __ L __ Finkelstein Test (De Quervain)	R __ L __ Talar Tilt
R __ L __ Tinel _____	R __ L __ Homan's
R __ L __ Phalen's	R __ L __ Thompson (Achilles tendon)
R __ L __ Bowstring (Biceps Tendon)	R __ L __ Other: _____

Assessment: _____

STGs (____ Weeks)
- ☐ Decrease Pain _____
- ☐ Increase ROM _____
- ☐ Decrease Edema _____
- ☐ Improve Postural Awareness _____
- ☐ Improve Gait/Stair Negotiation _____
- ☐ Improve Body Mechanics: _____
- ☐ I with HEP
- ☐ Other _____

LTGs (____ Weeks)
- ☐ Decrease Pain _____
- ☐ Increased ROM _____
- ☐ Increase Strength _____
- ☐ Postural Awareness _____
- ☐ Improved Gait/Stair Negotiation _____
- ☐ Return to Driving
- ☐ Return to Work
- ☐ Independent with ADLs _____

Plan of Treatment:
- ☐ Postural Education
- ☐ Work Station Ergonomics
- ☐ Ultrasound _____
- ☐ Mechanical Traction (Pt's wgt # _____)
- ☐ Therapeutic Exercise
- ☐ Taping

- ☐ Lifting Mechanics _____
- ☐ Electrical Stimulation _____
- ☐ Iontophoresis _____
- ☐ Heat/Ice _____
- ☐ Gait Training
- ☐ Manual Techniques _____

Frequency: _____x Per Week for _____ Weeks/Months

Rehabilitation Potential: ☐ Good   ☐ Fair   ☐ Poor

☐ Goals Discussed with Patient and Patient Expresses Understanding of Treatment Plan

Additional Comments: _____
_____
_____

Therapist Signature: _____ Date: _____

☐	Samuel H. Esterson, PT	Maryland License # 14937	Exp Date: 5/31/07
☐	Audra R. Stern, PT	Maryland License # 20006	Exp Date: 5/31/06
☐	Laura Reitman, PT	Maryland License # 18305	Exp Date: 5/31/07
☐	Karen Gordes, PT	Maryland License # 19269	Exp Date: 5/31/07

Medical History Questionnaire

ESTERSON & ASSOCIATES PHYSICAL THERAPY
MEDICAL HISTORY QUESTIONNAIRE

The purpose of this questionnaire is to help us understand your health status. Please complete this form and your therapist will answer any questions during your exam. This form is considered part of your medical record.

Name: _____ D.O.B./Age _____/_____

Referring Physician: _____ Family Physician: _____

Emergency Contact Name: _____ Phone:_____Cell:_____

Date of Last General Health Check-up _____/_____/_____ Occupation: _____

Last Date Worked Due to this Injury: _____/_____/_____ Date Returned to Work After This Injury: _____/_____/____

Have you had Surgery for this Injury?   YES   NO   Type of Surgery/Dates: _____

Is an Attorney Involved in this Case?   YES   NO Attorney Name: _____

Pain (please draw a vertical line where you would rate your pain intensity): 0------------------5------------------10
                                                                    No pain   Maximum Pain Tolerable
My pain can be described as: (please circle all that apply):
        Constant   Intermittent   Sharp   Dull   Aching   Stabbing   Numbness   Pins/Needles

Are You Currently Taking Any Prescription or Non-Prescription Medications?   YES   NO
        Anti-Inflammatories   Muscle Relaxers   Pain Medicines   Others: _____

Have you had any of the following Medical or Rehabilitative Care for this Injury/Episode? If yes, when? _____

	YES	NO		YES	NO
Chiropractor	___	___	CT Scan	___	___
General Practitioner	___	___	EMG/NCV	___	___
Occupational Therapy	___	___	MRI	___	___
Physical Therapy	___	___	Myelogram	___	___
Massage Therapy	___	___	X-Rays	___	___
Neurologist	___	___	Emergency Room Care	___	___
Orthopedist	___	___	Podiatrist	___	___

Do you now have, or have you ever had, any of the following?

	YES	NO		YES	NO
Asthma, Bronchitis, or Emphysema	___	___	Severe or Frequent Headaches	___	___
Shortness of Breath/Chest Pain	___	___	Vision or Hearing difficulty	___	___
Coronary Heart Disease or Angina	___	___	Numbness or Tingling	___	___
Do you have a Pacemaker	___	___	Dizziness or Fainting	___	___
High Blood Pressure	___	___	Weakness	___	___
Heart Attack/Heart Surgery	___	___	Weight Loss/Energy Loss	___	___
Blood Clot/Emboli	___	___	Hernia	___	___
Stroke/TIA	___	___	Epilepsy/Seizures	___	___
Allergies	___	___	Thyroid Trouble/Goiter	___	___
Pins or Metal Implants	___	___	Incontinence	___	___
Joint Replacement (any joint)	___	___	Bowel or Bladder Problems	___	___
Diabetes	___	___	Neck Injury/Surgery	___	___
Infectious Diseases	___	___	Shoulder Injury/Surgery	___	___
Cancer/Chemotherapy/Radiation	___	___	Elbow/Hand Injury/Surgery	___	___
Arthritis/Swollen Joints	___	___	Back Injury/Surgery	___	___
Osteoporosis	___	___	Knee Injury/Surgery	___	___
Sleeping Problems/Difficulty	___	___	Leg/Ankle/Foot Injury/Surgery	___	___
Do you smoke?	___	___	Multiple Sclerosis/Parkinson's	___	___
Latex Sensitivity/Allergy	___				

FOR WOMEN ONLY:	YES	NO		YES	NO
Pelvic inflammatory disease	___	___	Endometriosis	___	___
Irregular Menstrual Cycle	___	___	Incontinence (urinary/fecal)	___	___
Complicated pregnancies/deliveries?	___	___	Are you pregnant?	___	___

Patient/Guardian Signature: _____Date:_____

PT Initials _____ Date: _____

Patient Sign-In Sheet

Date: _____

Patient Name	Appt Time	Patient Name	Appt Time

Assignment of Benefits Form

PATIENT AGREEMENT TO ASSIGN
HEALTH CARE BENEFITS TO PROVIDER

In reference to payment outstanding for treatment of my injuries caused by my accident/trauma that occurred on or about _____ for which I have received physical therapy at Anyone's Physical Therapy Group, hereafter referred to as *'provider'*, located at Two West Anywhere Avenue, Suite # 100, Any City, Any State, 21228:

I, _____, hereafter referred as *'patient'*, hereby authorize and direct my attorney, _____, to fully compensate provider for any and all outstanding monies due provider at the time of settlement, financial award, court verdict, jury verdict, or arbitration, within ten days from the receipt of such an award, prior to attorney delivering funds from said settlement to me.

By my signature below, the patient guarantees that his/her attorney listed above, will pay within ten days of a financial settlement, financial award, court verdict, jury verdict, or arbitration, monies due Anyone's Physical Therapy Group as a result of injuries received from the aforementioned accident.

By my signature below, the attorney guarantees that he will forward monies directly upon receipt of financial award, court verdict, jury verdict, or arbitration, due Anyone's Physical Therapy Group stemming from fees associated with rendering care to the patient as a result of injuries incurred in aforementioned accident, within ten days of settlement. A monthly penalty of 7% will be added to the amount due provider should monies not be received by provider within ten days of aforementioned award/settlement.

The attorney incurs no liability for payments to the provider and shall not be responsible for any actions on the part of the patient that violate or seek to avoid the patient's obligation to compensate the provider.

The patient has the right to revoke the power of attorney at any time with proper notice to the provider, Anyone's Physical Therapy Group, address above.

The provider retains the right to terminate services if the patient revokes the power of attorney at any time prior to full payment of services rendered. Failure or refusal of patient and/or attorney to enter into this agreement is grounds for refusal of service by provider.

I fully understand and accept the terms and conditions of this agreement.

_____   _____
Anyone's Physical Therapy Group   Date

_____   _____
Patient   Date

_____   _____
Attorney   Date

Fax Cover Sheet

Anyone's Physical Therapy
Two West Anywhere Avenue • Suite 100 • Any City, Any State 21228
Phone (410) 747-2000 • FAX (410) 747-2002
www.yourtherapypractice.com

FAX COVER PAGE

TO: _____

FAX NUMBER: _____

FROM: _____

RE: _____

Total Number of Pages Sent (Including Cover Page): _____

THIS MESSAGE IS INTENDED ONLY FOR OFFICIAL BUSINESS USE BY THE INDIVIDUAL OR ENTITY TO WHICH IT IS ADDRESSED.

This fax may contain information that is privileged, confidential, and exempt from disclosure under applicable law. If the reader of this message is not the intended recipient, or the employee or agent responsible for delivery of the message to the intended recipient, you are hereby notified that any dissemination, distribution, or copying of this communication is strictly prohibited. If you have received this communication in error, please destroy this fax and notify the sender so that we may correct our records.

Physical Therapy Prescription Pad

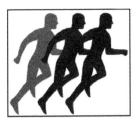

EJTERJON & AJJOCIATEJ
PHYJICAL THERAPY, P.A.
Two West Rolling Crossroads ◆ Suite 102
Baltimore, Maryland 21228
410.747.1600 ◆ Fax 410.747.5202
www.EstersonTherapy.com

R̶x PHYSICAL THERAPY

Patient's Name _____ Date _____

Dx: _____

Area/Part To Be Treated:_____

Precautions: _____ WB Status: _____

Evaluate and treat as appropriate ☐

Frequency   1   2   3   4   5   / week   Duration _____ weeks

I hereby certify that these services are medically necessary for the patient's plan of care.

Physician's Signature _____ Date _____

UPIN #_____ Email or fax # to contact referring physician _____

TREATMENT PROCEDURES:

☐ Mechanical Traction	☐ Therapeutic Exercise
☐ Cervical	☐ Passive
☐ Lumbar	☐ Active
☐ Hot/Cold Packs	☐ Resistive
☐ Iontophoresis	☐ Myofascial Release
☐ Ultrasound	☐ Desensitization
☐ Massage/Soft Tissue Work	☐ Paraffin Bath
☐ Home Exercise Program	☐ Manual Therapy
☐ Balance & Coordination Training	☐ Gait Training
☐ Intermittent Compression	☐ Isokinetic Testing
☐ Work Hardening Program	☐ Joint Mobilization
☐ Urinary Incontinence Program	☐ TMJ Program
☐ Post-Partum Program	☐ Electrical Stimulation
☐ Other: _____	

☐ Doctor: Please check here if more referral pads are needed

DIRECTIONS FROM THE BELTWAY: Exit 17 Security Boulevard towards Rolling Road. After three
traffic lights turn left on Rolling Road. Pass three short traffic lights and see our building complex on your
left. We are in the West Building. Look for the large **PHYSICAL THERAPY** sign over our entry doors.

Notice of Patient Information Practices

THIS NOTICE DESCRIBES HOW MEDICAL AND PERSONAL INFORMATION ABOUT YOU MAY BE USED OR DISCLOSED AND HOW YOU CAN OBTAIN ACCESS TO THIS INFORMA-TION. PLEASE REVIEW THIS FORM CAREFULLY.

OUR LEGAL DUTY
Anyone's Physical Therapy, P.A. is required by law to protect the privacy of your personal and health information, provide notice about our information management practices, and follow the information protocols described below.

USES AND DISCLOSURES OF HEALTH INFORMATION
Anyone's Physical Therapy, P.A. uses your personal and health information primarily for treatment, obtaining payment for treatment, conducting internal administrative activities, and assessing the quality of care we are proud to provide. We use your personal information to contact you to arrange an appointment with us and to properly bill your insurance carrier for the services we provide you with. In addition, we may, from time to time, disclose your health information without prior authorization for public health purposes, auditing tracking, and research studies. In any other situation, Anyone's Physical Therapy, P.A. will obtain your written permission and authorization before disclosing your personal health information. If you provide us with written authorization to release your information for any reason, you may later revoke that authorization to cease future disclosures at any time. If and when any changes are made in our privacy and confidentiality policies, a new Notice of Information Practices will be posted in the same area for public view. You may request a copy of our Notice of Information Practices at any time. Our HIPAA Compliance Officer is Sandra Joe. She can be reached at the office by calling (410) 747-2000.

PATIENT'S INDIVIDUAL RIGHTS
You have the right to review or obtain a copy of your personal health information at any time. You have the right to request that we correct inaccurate or incomplete information in your records. You also have the right to request a list of instances where we disclosed your personal health information for reasons other than for treatment, payment, or other related administrative purposes. You may request in writing that we not use or disclose your personal health information for treatment, payment, or administrative purposes except when specifically authorized by you, when required by law, or in an emergency. Anyone's Physical Therapy, P.A. will consider all such requests on a case-by-case basis. The company is not legally required to accept the requests.

CONCERNS AND COMPLAINTS
If you are concerned that Anyone's Physical Therapy, P.A. may have violated your privacy rights or if you disagree with any decisions we have made regarding access or disclosure of your personal health information, please contact our HIPAA Compliance Officer, Sandra Joe, at the office address and phone number listed below. You may also send a written complaint to the U.S. Department of Health and Human Services.

> Anyone's Physical Therapy, P.A.
> HIPAA Compliance Office
> Attention: Sandra Joe
> Two Oak Street
> Anytown, Any State 21228
> (410)747-2000

Every Patient Must Receive a Copy of This Form

Release of Records Form

Date: _____

By my signature below, I hereby authorize release of my medical records to Anyone's Physical Therapy, P.A.

Patient Name: _____

Date of Birth: _____

Records related to: _____

Patient's Signature: _____

Please fax records to:

Anyone's Physical Therapy, P.A.
Fax Number (410) 747-2002

Two West Anywhere Ave • Suite 100 • Anywhere, Any State 21228
Phone (410) 747-2000 • Fax (410) 747-2002

Appendix 13

Sample Employee Handbook Table of Contents Outline

INTRODUCTION

Mission Statement
About Us

EMPLOYMENT POLICIES
Equal Opportunity Employment
Immigration Law
Maryland New Hire Registry
COBRA
At Will Employment Relationship
Minimum Age Requirement
Employee Status
Probationary Period
Employee Evaluations
Standards of Conduct
Disciplinary Actions
Notice of Resignation
Personnel Files
Hours of Operation
Work Week
Overtime

WORK POLICIES
CPR Certification
TB Testing
Hepatitis-B Vaccination
HIPAA Policies
Schedules

Sign In Sheets
Absences
Late Arrival
Work Injuries
Staff Meetings
Uniform/Dress Code
Employee Grievances
Equipment/Office Supply Use
Leave of Absence
Maternity Leave
Continuing Education Leave
Jury Duty
Voting
Wage Confidentiality
Inclement Weather
Personal Phone Calls
Smoking
Parking
Safety and Security
Duties Prior to Daily Close

BENEFITS
Vacation
Sick Leave
Holidays
Health Insurance
Dental Insurance
Life Insurance
Waiver of Insurance Coverage

APPENDICES
Employee Acknowledgment Form
Group Health Insurance Coverage Waiver Form
Deferral of Hepatitis Vaccination Series

Appendix 14

Sample Employment Agreement

This employment Agreement ("Agreement") is made on _____ _____
_____ _____ by and between Anyone's Physical
Therapy (Employer) and _____
(Employee) of 123 Any Road, Any Town, Any State 21228.

    A. Employer is engaged in the business of physical therapy services.

    B. Employer desires to have the services of the employee.

    C. Employee is willing to be employed by employer.

        1. Employment. Employer shall employ employee as a staff therapist to render physical therapy services to the practice's private patients as well as to patients at the various contract facilities. Employee accepts and agrees to such employment subject to the general supervision, advice, and direction of employer and the employer's supervisory personnel. Employee shall also perform (i) such other duties as are customarily performed by an employee in a similar position, and (ii) such other and unrelated services and duties as may be assigned to the employee from time to time by the employer.

        2. Best Efforts of Employee. Employee agrees to perform faithfully, industriously, and to the best of employee's abilities, experience and talents, all of the duties that may be required by the express and implicit terms of this Agreement, to the reasonable satisfaction of the employer. Such duties shall be provided at Anytown, Maryland and at such other place(s) as the needs, business, or opportunities of the employer may require from time to time.

        3. Compensation of Employee. As compensation for the services provided by the employee under this agreement, employer will pay employee a sum of $ _____ per hour. This amount shall be paid in accordance with the regulations set forth in

the practice's Employee Handbook. Upon termination of this Agreement, payments under this paragraph shall cease; provided, however, that the employee shall be entitled to payments for periods or partial periods that occurred prior to the date of termination and for which the employee has not yet been paid.

4. Reimbursement for Expenses in Accordance with Employer Policy. The employer will reimburse employee for "out-of-pocket" expenses in accordance with the employer's policies as set out in the Employee Handbook.

5. Termination Due to Discontinuance of Business. Should the employer discontinue operations, this Agreement shall terminate upon notice as provided in this Agreement.

6. Recommendations for Improving Operations. Employee shall provide employer all information regarding employer's business of which employee has knowledge. Employee shall make all suggestions and recommendations that will be of mutual benefit to employer and employee.

7. Confidentiality. Employee recognizes that employer has and will have business affairs, future plans, prices, customer lists, technical information, costs, and other vital information (collectively Information), which are valuable, special, and proprietary assets belonging to the employer. Employee agrees that employee will not, at any time or in any manner, either directly or indirectly, disclose, divulge, or communicate in any manner any information to any third party without the prior written consent of the employer. Employee will protect the information and treat it as strictly confidential. A violation by employee of this paragraph shall be a material violation of this agreement and will justify legal and/or equitable relief and remedy.

   a. Unauthorized Disclosure of Information. If it appears that employee has disclosed (or has threatened to disclose) information in violation of this agreement, employer shall be entitled to an injunction to restrain employee from disclosing, in whole or in part, such information, or from providing any services to any party to whom such information has been disclosed or may be disclosed. Employer shall not be prohibited from pursuing other remedies, including a claim for loss and damage.

b. Confidentiality after Termination of Employment. The confidentiality provisions of this agreement shall remain in full force and effect for a period of two years after the termination of employee's employment.

8. Employee's Inability to Contract for Employer. Employee shall not have the right to make any contracts or commitments for or on behalf of employer without first obtaining the express, written consent of the employer.

9. Vacation, Sick Leave, Holidays, Health and Life Insurance Plans, Pension Plan, and Other Benefits. As a full-time, permanent member of the staff, employee is eligible for benefits as set forth in the Employee Handbook. Employee will be notified in writing as to any changes made by employer to employee benefits.

10. Term and Termination. Employee's employment under this agreement shall be for one year, beginning on _____. This agreement may be terminated by either party upon four weeks' written notice. If employee is in violation of this agreement or any portion of the practice code of conduct as set forth in the Employee Handbook, employer may terminate employment immediately without notice and with compensation to employee only to the date of such termination.

11. Termination for Disability. Employer shall have the option to terminate this agreement if employee becomes permanently disabled. Employer shall exercise this option by giving 14 days' written notice to employee. For the purposes of this agreement, employee shall be deemed permanently disabled if employee is unable to perform substantially all of his/her duties for a period of time in excess of 90 days because of ill health, physical or mental disability, or for other causes beyond employee's control.

12. Compliance with Employer's Rules. Employee agrees to submit to all of the rules and regulations of employer in this contract, future mutually executed documents, and the Employee Handbook.

13. Return of Records. Upon termination of this agreement, employee shall deliver all property (including keys, records, notes, data, memoranda, models, and equipment) that is in the employee's possession or under the employee's control that is

employer's property or related to employee's business by the final date of the employee's employment.

14. Notices. All notices as required or permitted under this agreement shall be in writing and shall be deemed delivered when delivered in person or deposited in the United States mail, postage paid, addressed as follows:

> To Employer: Any Employer
> Attention: Any Owner
> 123 Any Road
> Any City, Any State 21228
>
> To Employee: Any Employee
> 567 Employee Road
> Any Town, Any State 21228

Such addresses may be changed from time-to-time by either party by providing written notice in the manner set forth above.

15. Entire Agreement. This agreement contains the entire agreement of the parties and there are no other promises or conditions in any other agreement whether oral or written. This agreement supercedes any prior written or oral agreements between the parties.

16. Amendment. This agreement may be modified or amended if amendment is made in writing and is signed by both parties.

17. Severability. If any provision of this agreement shall be held to be invalid or unenforceable for any reason, the remaining provisions shall continue to be valid and enforceable. If a court finds that any provision of this agreement is invalid or unenforceable, but that by limiting such provision it would become valid and enforceable, then such provision shall be deemed to be written, construed, and enforced as so limited.

18. Waiver of Contractual Right. The failure of either party to enforce any provision of this agreement shall not be construed as a waiver or limitation of that party's right to subsequently enforce and compel strict compliance with every provision of this agreement.

19. Applicable State Law. This agreement shall be governed by the laws of the State of _____.
    Agreed this _____ day of _____, 20 _____.

By:_____, PT President

By:_____, Employee

Appendix 15

Resources for Further Information on Private Physical Therapy Practice

- Private Practice Section of the American Physical Therapy Association. Business law, strategic planning, human resources issues, and general preparation for success for private practitioners: *http://www.ppsapta.org/*

- Building a Private Practice: Tools, resources, general information analysis spreadsheets by Peter Kovacek: *http://ptmanager.com/starting_a_new_therapy_practice.htm*

- Summary of the P.T. in Private Practice Medicare Enrollment Process: *http://www.apta.org/Govt_Affairs/regulatory/privatepractice/ general_requiremts/view15*

- Reimbursement Issues, Government Affairs, and general information for clinicians: *http://www.apta.org/reimbursement*

- Advance for Physical Therapists. Professional newsletter that advises more than 100,000 healthcare practitioners and specializes in the design and implementation of private practice growth and marketing: *http://www.advanceforpt.com/pt.html*

- Discussion forums, journal articles, and more, by David Adamczyk, MS, PT, and Randy Moore, MS, PT: *http://www.private-practice.com/*

- HIPAA resources as they relate to physical therapy: *http://www.ptwa.org/HIPAA.htm* *http://www.hipaadvisory.com/regs/* *http://www.cms.hhs.gov/hipaa/hipaa2/regulations/lsnotify.asp*

- U.S. Small Business Administration: *http://www.sba.gov/*

- Site for small business questions and answers: *http://www.bizoffice.com/*

- The online small business authority with information to help you start, grow, or manage your small business: *http://www.entrepreneur.com/*

- Sample contracts, letters of intent, consulting agreements, and others: *http://www.allbusiness.com/*

- Human Resources management and advice: *http://www.business.com/ directory/human_resources/hiring_and_retention/index.asp*

- Starting and managing a small business: *http://www.morebusiness.com/*

- Consumer Health Educational Council: *www.healthchec.org*

- National Council of Insurance Commissioners: *www.naic.org*

- U.S. Census Bureau: *www.census.gov/hhes/www/hlthins.html*

- American Association of Health Plans: *www.aahp.org*

- Compliance issues, fraud, and abuse: *www.ppsapta.org*

- Books and periodicals online: *www.Amazon.com*

- Managed Care Reference list and other guides through the APTA's Section on Administration: *www.aptasoa.org*

Appendix 16

State Insurance Carrier List Example (State of Maryland)

PARTICIPATING CARRIERS

Aetna Life Insurance Company
151 Farmington Avenue
Hartford, CT 06156
410-691-1080

Aetna Health, Inc.
1301 McCormick Drive
Largo, MD 20774
1-301-636-0000

CareFirst BlueChoice, Inc.
550 12th Street, SW
Washington, DC 20065
1-202-479-8000

CareFirst of MD, Inc.
10455 Mill Run Circle
Owings Mills, MD 21117
1-800-537-5963

Cigna Healthcare Mid-Atlantic, Inc.
Attn: Rena Mojecki
7125 Columbia Gateway Drive
Columbia, MD 21046
1-443-259-6156

Coventry Health & Life, Inc.
2751 Centerville Road
Suite 400
Wilmington, DE 19808
1-800-727-9951, ext. 1144

Coventry Healthcare of Delaware, Inc.
2751 Centerville Road
Suite 400
Wilmington, DE 19808
1-800-727-9951, ext. 1144

Fidelity Insurance Company
201 International Circle, 4th Floor
Hunt Valley, MD 21030
410-329-0900

Graphic Arts Benefit Corporation
6411 Ivy Lane, Suite 700
Greenbelt, MD 20770
1-800-469-1673

Group Hospitalization & Medical Services
Trading as CareFirst BlueCross BlueShield
550 12th Street, SW
Washington, DC 20065
1-202-479-8000

Guardian Life Insurance Co. of America
Small Group Sales (groups with 15 or fewer)
3900 Burgess Place
Bethlehem, PA 18017
1-800-356-5808

Guardian Life Insurance Co. of America
MidAtlantic Group Sales Office (more than 15)
11785 Beltsville Drive, Suite 1200
Calverton Five Flagship Building
Beltsville, MD 20705
1-800-945-6584 or 1-301-586-1500

**Kaiser Foundation Health Plan of the
Mid-Atlantic States, Inc.**
2101 East Jefferson Street
PO Box 6611
Rockville, MD 20849-6611
1-443-663-6181 or 1-703-873-1500

MAMSI Life & Health Insurance Company
4 Taft Court
Rockville, MD 20850
1-800-709-7604

MEGA Life & Health Insurance Company
PO Box 982010
North Richland Hills, TX 76182
1-800-527-5504

**Mid-West National Life Insurance Company of
Tennessee**
PO Box 982010
North Richland Hills, TX 76182
1-800-733-1110

Optimum Choice, Inc.
4 Taft Court
Rockville, MD 20850
1-800-709-7604

PHN-HMO, Inc.
Airport Square
1099 Winterson Road
Linthicum, MD 21090-2216
410-850-7461

United HealthCare Insurance Company
4416 East West Highway
Suite 310
Bethesda, MD 20814
1-866-297-9264

Source: www.mdinsurance.state.md.us/

Appendix 17

Opening Day Checklist

With clipboard in hand, the following checklist should be completed prior to the arrival of your first patient:

☐ All your treatment and safety equipment should be assembled and in place.

☐ Remove all clutter and store soft goods in a user-friendly manner.

☐ Linens and table covering (sheets or table paper) should be laundered and in place.

☐ Your staff, no matter how meager, should be familiar with the intake procedure that you have set up.

☐ Staff must be familiar with emergency and evacuation procedures.

☐ Staff must be knowledgeable of privacy and security issues as they relate to HIPAA regulations.

☐ The front office should be prepared with the necessary forms for collecting the proper information you require for billing and recordkeeping purposes.

☐ Chart folders and filing systems should be ready and in place.

☐ Insurance provider and contact numbers should be posted and accessible to staff.

☐ Evaluation and encounter forms, pens, evaluation tools (goniometers, reflex hammers, etc.) should be ready for the initial evaluation and treatment.

☐ Telephones, fax machine, and copy machine should be ready and in working order.

☐ Business and appointment cards should be available for scheduling the patient's next visit.

☐ Receipt book should be available to provide patient with receipt for co-pay, if needed.

Appendix 18
Wise Words Author Listing

- **Thomas Jefferson** was the third president of the United States from 1801–1809. He was eloquent as a writer and a correspondent, but he was no public speaker. In the Virginia House of Burgesses and the Continental Congress, he contributed his pen rather than his voice toward the fight for independence. As the "silent member" of the Congress, Jefferson, at 33, drafted the Declaration of Independence. In the years following, he labored to make its words a reality in Virginia. Most notably, he wrote a bill establishing religious freedom, enacted in 1786. He was born on April 13, 1743 in Albermarle County, Virginia and died on July 4, 1826 at Monticello in Virginia.

- **Albert Einstein** was born on March 14, 1879, in Germany. He grew up in Munich, where his father owned a small electrochemical factory. The strict discipline of German schools did not appeal to the young Einstein, who was a poor student, but he independently studied philosophy, math, and science. He taught himself calculus and higher scientific principles. After failing his first entrance examination to the prestigious Swiss Federal Institute of Technology in Zurich, Einstein gained admittance in 1896 and began his four years studying physics and mathematics. After his graduation in 1900, Einstein became a naturalized Swiss citizen in 1901 and got a job as a technical assistant at the Swiss patent office in Bern. In 1903, he married his university sweetheart, Mileva Maric. While employed at the patent office, Einstein continued his own investigations in theoretical physics. Einstein received the Nobel Prize in 1921 for his work on the photoelectric effect. He is remembered as a brilliant scientist and great thinker.

- **Frank Lloyd Wright** was born in 1867 and died in 1957. He is considered to be one of the most influential architects of our time, designing over 1,000 structures, of which about 400 were built. He described his "organic architecture" as one that "proceeds, persists, and creates, according to the nature of man and his circumstances as they both change." As a pioneer whose ideas were well ahead of his time, Wright had to fight for acceptance of every new design. His style was influenced by his father's classical music and the building blocks his mother gave him. He was outspoken and creatively wrote as well.

- **Pearl (nee Sydenstricker) Buck**, born in 1892, was one of the most popular American authors of her day, noted for her rich and truly epic descriptions of peasant life in China and for her biographical masterpieces for which she was awarded the Nobel Prize for Literature in 1938. She was also a humanitarian, crusader for women's rights, and a philanthropist.

- **William Jennings Bryan** was a U.S. congressman, three-time Democratic presidential nominee, secretary of state, and was a major force in American politics for three decades. Bryan was born on March 19, 1860, in Salem, Illinois. He attended college, studied law, and entered legal practice in Illinois before moving to Lincoln, Nebraska, in 1887. When nominated for President for the second time, in 1900, Bryan insisted on a platform endorsing free silver but emphasized imperialism as a more important issue. In 1908 he won the Democratic presidential nomination for a third time but again lost the election. Bryan was a political evangelist. Often ahead of his time as a spokesman for liberal causes, he was also closely identified with traditionalism, particularly with Fundamentalist Christianity.

- **Carl Jung** (1875–1961) was a Swiss-German psychiatrist who, with Sigmund Freud, was instrumental in bringing psychology into the twentieth century. Jung developed a ground-breaking personality theory that introduced the world to the concepts of extraversion and introversion and explained human behavior as a combination of four psychic functions—thinking, feeling, intuition, and sensation. He is credited as the founder of analytical psychology. He is perhaps best known for postulating the collective unconscious, those acts and mental patterns shared universally by all human beings. He wrote extensively on psychoanalysis and human behavior.

- **Jonathan Swift** was born in Dublin, Ireland in 1667. He was a prolific writer and satirist and was best known for his popular book, *Gulliver's Travels*. Though it's been described as a children's book, it is also a great satire of the times in which he lived. Upon deeper study, the book describes Gulliver's tall tales with current events and long-term societal problems.

- **Sandra Day O'Connor** is the first female member of the United States Supreme Court. She was born in 1930 in El Paso, Texas and grew up on her family's 198,000-acre cattle ranch. She is a 1952 graduate of the Stanford Law School and, after she married, served as an Arizona assistant attorney general from 1965 to 1969, when she was appointed to a vacancy in the Arizona Senate. In 1974, she ran successfully for trial judge, a position she held until she was appointed to the Arizona Court of Appeals in 1979. Eighteen months later, on July 7, 1981, President Ronald Reagan nominated her to the Supreme Court. In September 1981, Sandra Day O'Connor became the Court's 102nd justice and its first female member. Her votes are generally conservative, but she frequently surprises observers with her political independence.

- **Dwight Morrow**'s claim to fame was not that he was the United States Ambassador to Mexico in the 1920s, but rather that his daughter, Anne, married Charles Lindbergh, the famous American solo flyer across the Atlantic Ocean. Mr. Morrow was a politician whose service was notable because it marked a new spirit of cooperation in U.S. relations with Latin America. Following his Ambassadorship, he served (1930–31) in the U.S. Senate as a Republican from New Jersey.

- **George Bernard Shaw** was born in 1856. He grew up to become an active Socialist and a brilliant platform speaker, writing on many social aspects of the day. He was a famous playwright and a witty essayist who won the Nobel Prize in the early 1990s. He died in 1950.

- **Benjamin Disraeli** lived from 1804 through 1881 and was known as a very sharp-witted novelist, a brilliant debater, and England's first and only Jewish prime minister. He is best remembered for bringing India and the Suez Canal under control of the crown. Disraeli was elected to Parliament in 1837 after failing to win a seat in four earlier elections.

- **Hannah Senesh** was born in Hungary in 1921, the daughter of a prominent Jewish playwright. She exhibited a precocious writing talent and remarkable intelligence. Hannah lived a typical upper-middle class life until age 17 when she became involved in the Zionist movement to create a Jewish state in Palestine. Emigrating there in 1939, she worked on a kibbutz until 1943 when Hannah joined the Jewish underground and enlisted in the British Army. After receiving a commission and training in a parachuting unit, Hannah was captured in Hungary on a mission to rescue Jews and send information via radio. Held prisoner, tortured, and finally executed, Hannah was barely 23.

- **Bill Cosby** is an award winning actor, writer, educator, comedian, TV/radio host, producer, and composer. He was born William H. Cosby Jr. on July 12, 1937 in Philadelphia, Pennsylvania. He is one of the most influential stars in America today. Whether it be through concert appearances or recordings, television or films, commercials or education, Bill Cosby has the ability to touch people's lives. He tickles his audiences by openly discussing family relationships, work, and life in general. He is one of the most recognizable names in entertainment today.

- **Rudyard Kipling** (1865–1936) was born in Bombay and educated in England. He was primarily known as a writer of short stories. A prolific writer, he achieved fame quickly. Kipling was the poet of the British Empire and its yeoman, the common soldier, whom he glorified in many of his works. In 1907, he was the recipient of the Nobel Prize for Literature.

- **Ralph Waldo Emerson** was born in Boston in 1803 and educated at Harvard. He initially dedicated his life to serving as a minister in the Unitarian Church of Boston, but eventually left the pulpit to pursue a career in public speaking and writing. He was an inspiration for many writers, especially Henry Thoreau and Walt Whitman. Emerson became one of America's best known and best loved 19th century figures. He died in 1882.

About the Author

Samuel Esterson is a licensed physical therapist with over 20 years experience working in many practice venues. From corporate to consulting, academia to private entrepreneurship, and mentor to hospital staff therapist, he has always aimed to get the most of his position, learning new and important things along the way. He is a driven man, always aiming for higher goals in practice and life in general. The author's most recent pursuit, that of earning his clinical doctorate in physical therapy, took him to the University of Maryland School of Medicine, Department of Physical Therapy and Rehabilitation Sciences, where he was a proud member of its first graduating class. Dr. Esterson earned a bachelor's degree in physical therapy in 1979 and upon graduation took a position at the Rusk Institute of Rehabilitation Medicine in New York City. Dr. Esterson credits Rusk with teaching him the basics of clinical care and management, as well as offering him the possibility of attending New York University where, under the tutelage of Dr. Marilyn Moffat and Dr. Arthur Nelson, two of the profession's leading academics, he earned a master's degree in pathokinesiology, the study of abnormal human motion. Over the years, Dr. Esterson worked in outpatient facilities and finally settled down into working with an established private practice group in the Washington, DC suburbs. Dr. Esterson gleaned as much business education as he could from his mentors there, finally opening his own private practice in Baltimore in 1985. As business became rocky in the mid 1990s, the author decided to sell his practice to a publicly held corporate entity, remaining on site as clinical manager for two more years. In 1997, he opted to take a year's sabbatical to return to school and study business administration. He attended Bar Ilan University in

Israel, earning an MBA in 1998. Upon return to Baltimore, Dr. Esterson was recruited to establish and manage a corporate-owned facility that he successfully grew until his most recent change of venue. The lure of private enterprise once again called Dr. Esterson, so in 2002 he reopened his own practice. It is growing exponentially with the use of the valuable information found in these pages.

Dr. Esterson and his wife, Malka, a registered nurse in the Baltimore County Public Schools, have been married for 22 years. They have three sons aged 18, 16, and 12.

Index